Sugar High

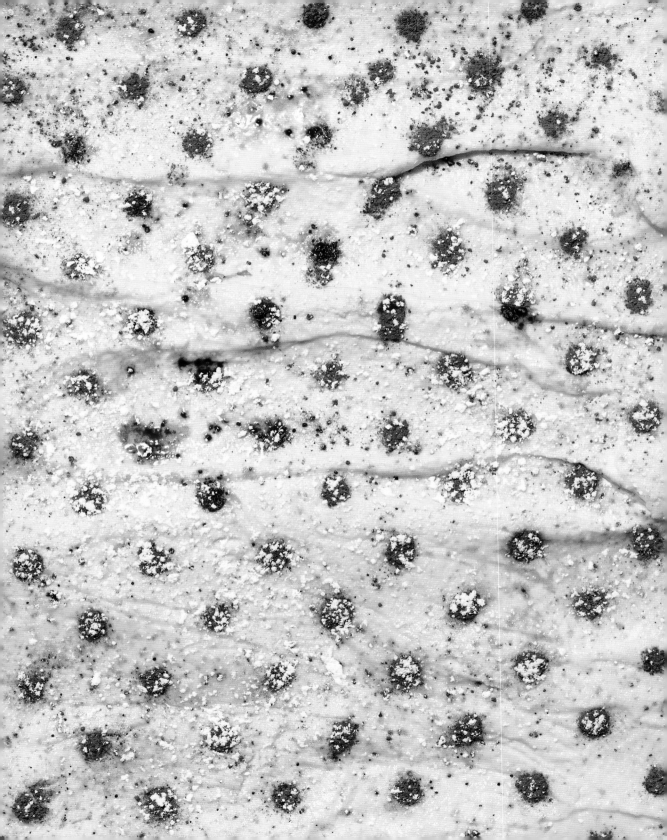

Chris Sayegh

SUGAR HIGH

50 RECIPES FOR CANNABIS DESSERTS

SIMON ELEMENT   NEW YORK   LONDON   TORONTO   SYDNEY   NEW DELHI

SIMON
ELEMENT

An Imprint of Simon & Schuster, Inc.
1230 Avenue of the Americas
New York, NY 10020

First Simon Element hardcover edition February 2023

SIMON ELEMENT and its colophon are trademarks of Simon & Schuster, Inc.

For information about special discounts for bulk purchases, please contact Simon & Schuster Special Sales at 1-866-506-1949 or business@simonandschuster.com.

The Simon & Schuster Speakers Bureau can bring authors to your live event. For more information or to book an event, contact the Simon & Schuster Speakers Bureau at 1-866-248-3049 or visit our website at www.simonspeakers.com.

Interior design by Matt Ryan
Photography produced by Blueline Creative Group LLC
Visit bluelinecreativegroup.com
Producer: Katherine Cobbs
Photographer: Caitlin Bensel
Food Stylist: Torie Cox
Food Stylist Assistant: Sally McKay
Prop Stylist: Mindi Shapiro
Prop Stylist Assistant: Brett Levine

Manufactured in China

1 3 5 7 9 10 8 6 4 2

Library of Congress Cataloging-in-Publication Data has been applied for.

ISBN 978-1-9821-8564-0
ISBN 978-1-9821-8566-4 (ebook)

I dedicate this book first and
foremost to all those who love
to create.

Secondly, to those who understand
the true nature of cannabis and its
ability to help heal humanity.

Lastly, I dedicate this book to all
those who have been incarcerated,
taken away from their lives, or
died to defend the sacredness of
this plant. Without you, I could not
be here representing our collective
beliefs.

Contents

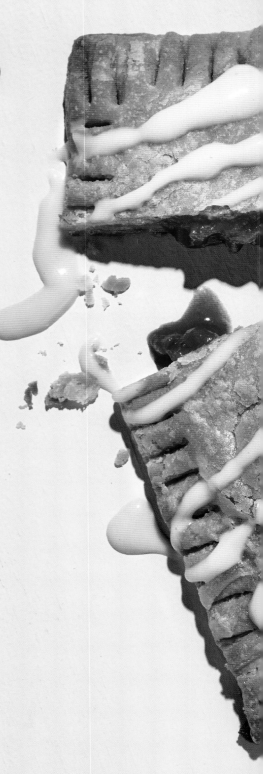

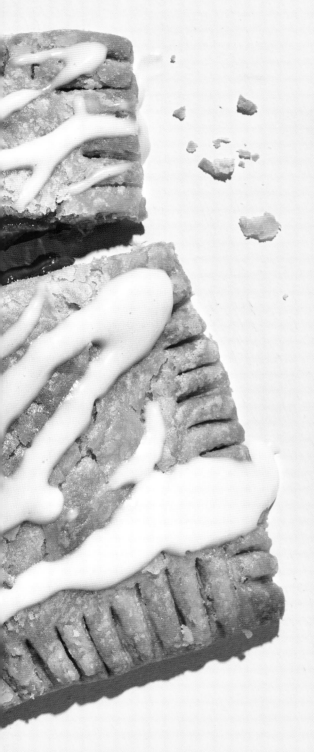

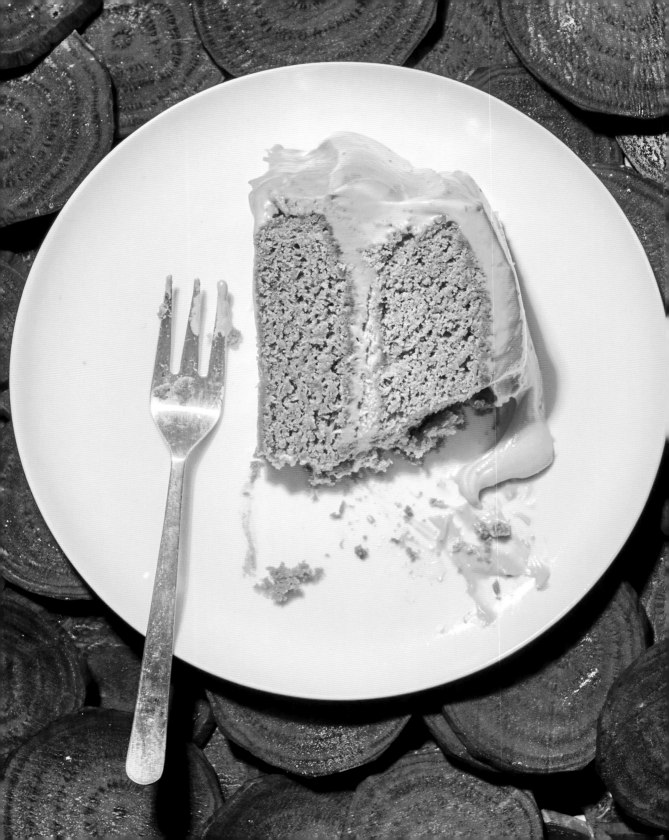

INTRODUCTION

If this is your first time purchasing anything even remotely cannabis-related, welcome. It's an honor to guide you through this journey. If you're a seasoned veteran and came solely for these bomb-ass recipes, I greet you with open arms and a moist cake, too.

Before we go too far into this cookbook, I want to explain a few things about what you will find here. First, you will learn why I love cannabis. I will also tell the story of cannabis: how and why it came to North America, its history, and its prevalence in today's society. Third, I will share with you why I treat cannabis with the utmost respect. It is an incredibly healing and overall versatile plant. Finally, this book was created with low-dose edibles in mind. I'll give you the tools to adjust recipes for the potency that's right for you.

I want to share my story. It begins when I moved to Northern California to attend the University of California Santa Cruz. That's where I fell in love with cannabis. My very first experience with cannabis had been in high school, and it was the classic, giggly high uninitiated people often experience. This was in 2010, and there were many cannabis strains to smoke, but the ready-made edibles were horrible. The only thing I could get my hands on were super bitter and grassy-tasting brownies and cereal treats. It felt more like I was eating weeds than dessert.

I knew there was a better way to enjoy edibles.

UCSC is a school of the sciences, which is ultimately why I chose to attend as a molecular cell biology major. What it doesn't say in the prospective student material is that Santa Cruz is also a place of exploration, including exploration of psychedelics and the mind. At Santa Cruz, I could openly study psychedelics without being judged. That alone sent my brain into overdrive. It led me to find my true life purpose, which is studying and understanding plant medicine. It has helped me achieve self-acceptance, sincere and authentic love, patience, and a feeling of peace I didn't know was possible. If this all feels a bit too far out there for you, then I will share with you a general understanding of what plant medicines and cannabis did for me: they helped me become the loving, caring, and dedicated man I am today.

The book you are holding represents years of research and recipe testing. The culmination of all of that hard work has made it possible for me to share my knowledge of cannabis, and to help destigmatize it as a serious and important medicinal herb, rather than just a means to getting high. I am confident that cooking with it can be life changing. It was for me.

It has been nearly a decade since I first started making edibles for my friends. At the time, I was beginning to suspect that cannabis had been getting a bad rap. After all, the plant has been used for centuries to promote health, but if I were caught with a joint I could go to jail. I started reading medical journals and papers that recounted how people had found healing in cannabis use. I felt like I had stumbled upon a holy grail that most of our contemporary civilization had missed.

In addition to my love affair with plants and herbs, I also have a crazy sweet tooth. And so, between those two passions, I felt I had an opportunity to erase all the misconceptions of cannabis if I could cook my way into people's hearts. *Sugar High* is a love letter to both cannabis and dessert.

Chocolate-forward recipes are abundant in this book because it's my absolute favorite flavor, but I've also included a variety of other desserts, too. I wanted to make sure that there was something for everyone, so you will also recognize a few nostalgic treats here, like cherry sherbet, apple pie, and brownies, but with my spin on them. Every recipe was developed with the average home cook in mind, and I've included a few challenging recipes in case you, too, want to impress yourself and please your friends with something unexpected.

With that, I introduce you to *Sugar High*.

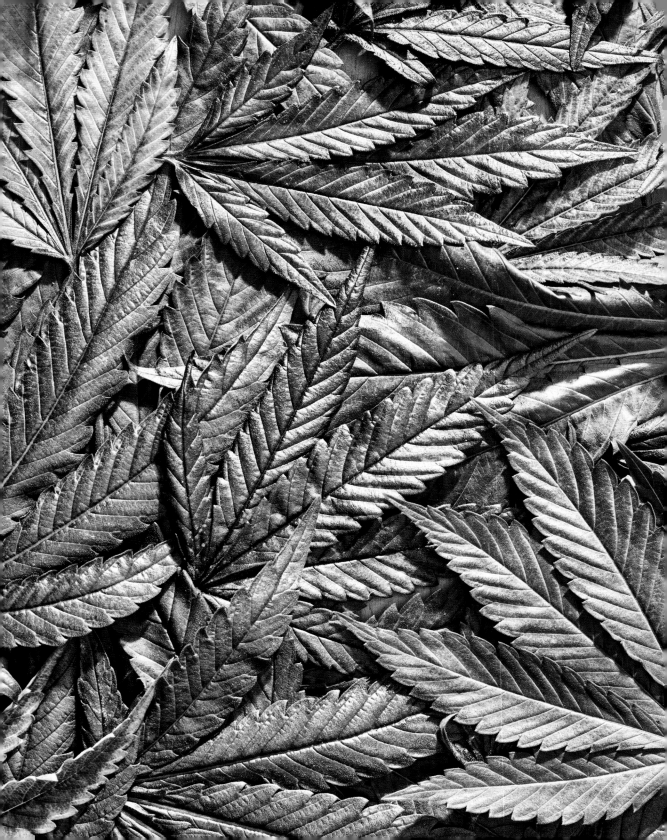

CHAPTER 1

UNDERSTANDING CANNABIS

While I've been asked countless questions regarding cannabis, the one I receive the most is "But *why use it*?" It's a valid question that I usually answer with the discussion of the herb's three main characteristics: the history of cannabis prohibition, hemp and its many uses, and the plant's medicinal components.

The History of Cannabis

Cannabis has been a huge part of daily life for most Eastern cultures since the beginning of recorded history. It grows practically everywhere (hence the name *weed*!). In early Western culture, it was used as a cure-all for almost every ailment. In fact, up until the early 1900s, it was found in many homeopathic and doctor-prescribed medications.

In traditional Chinese medicine, Emperor Shen Nung, known as the Father of Chinese Medicine, declared cannabis one of fifty fundamental herbs in his first published pharmacology book, *Pen ts'ao*, in 2737 BC. Shen Nung believed so much in its healing properties that he even accepted hemp as a form of payment. He prescribed hemp to help more than one hundred ailments, including gout, rheumatism, and even the absentmindedness that accompanies malaria.

Cannabis was used in Korea and India as early as 2000 BC and came to be known as *bhang*. Bhang's use was ubiquitous, and ranged from the rituals of spiritual ceremonies to decorative arts (such as pottery and making clothing). It was prized for its versatility and adaptability. A little later, cannabis appeared in Egyptian medical scrolls, where it was used to treat eye sores and cataracts. Cannabis pollen was found in the tomb of the mummified Ramesses II, the third pharaoh of the nineteenth dynasty of Egypt, suggesting that royalty was especially privy to the plant's healing powers.

In the Middle East, cannabis was a bit late to bloom. It was introduced around 1400 BC by nomadic Indo-European groups, and its medicinal use there was first recorded in 700 BC in the *Vendidad*, an ancient Persian text.

In the 1500s, the Spaniards introduced hemp to the Americas. By the early 1600s, cannabis came to Jamestown, where it became a cash crop; it was coveted for its use in making durable fabrics and sturdy dwellings. By the mid-seventeenth century, it even surpassed tobacco in profitability.

In the late nineteenth century, cannabis, which was easy to grow and seemingly effective as a medicine, started to threaten early industrialists who were profiting from pharmaceuticals. It was also increasingly used for recreation, and it was especially associated with the Mexican immigrants who came to the United States after the Mexican Revolution began in 1910. It's not hard to see what came next: between the threat to white industrialists' wallets and their proclivity to racism, by 1937, the US government had enacted the Marihuana Tax Act, effectively banning sales and distribution of cannabis. Just a year earlier, the propaganda film *Reefer Madness* had been released. It portrayed high schoolers committing heinous crimes while under the influence of marijuana. This was information warfare. When linked to use among Mexicans and other people of color for whom cannabis use was a centuries-old cultural tradition, cannabis became a catchall cause for everything from the Great Depression to unemployment to truancy. I believe, as do many of my colleagues in the cannabis industry, that the government knew the benefits of cannabis—financially, medicinally, and spiritually. Yet lawmakers were financially incentivized to lie to the public about the plant's capabilities and to demonize its use through the *Reefer Madness* campaign and the subsequent war on drugs that followed decades later. In the last fifty years, the federal government has spent $9.2 million *every single day* to incarcerate people on drug charges for owning a plant it arbitrarily maligned. And those people are mostly people of color, who are four times more likely than white people to be incarcerated for the same crime. It is as if they are being targeted.[1]

By 2003, the Department of Health and Human Services recognized the use of cannabinoids (which include THC, i.e., the psychoactive substance in cannabis) to help treat disease, such as Alzheimer's, cancer, diabetes, and neurodegenerative diseases caused by oxidative stress.[2] It takes a special kind of tyranny to say that something is unequivocally detrimental to people's well-being while also issuing a patent saying the opposite.

Cannabis as a Medicinal and Healthful Ingredient

CBD, which is just one compound of hundreds found in the cannabis plant, has been shown to effectively help numerous ailments and conditions, from insomnia and nausea (especially as a result of chemotherapy) to anxiety, pain, and life-threatening forms of epilepsy. Cannabis, however, is not just curative; it can also be preventative and part of a well-balanced diet. Hulled hemp seeds provide 64 percent of the daily value of protein per 100-gram serving. They are packed with amino acids, a rich source of B vitamins, and the hulled seed oil provides micronutrients and minerals, such as magnesium, phosphorus, zinc, iron, and fiber. And those are just the benefits of the actual seeds! The amino acid profile of the hemp seed is comparable to other, much less sustainable sources of protein, such as meat, milk, eggs, and soy. The overwhelming majority of energy provided by hemp seeds is in the form of fats and essential fatty acids, mainly polyunsaturated fatty acids and linoleic, oleic, and alpha-linolenic acids.

So when I'm asked "But *why use cannabis?*" the only answer that comes to mind is, *Why not?*

Diving into the Endocannabinoid System

There are more than one hundred kinds of cannabinoids (and counting!), but focusing on three makes for a strong introduction.

WHAT IS CBD?

CBD, or Cannabidiol, is a nonpsychoactive compound found in marijuana and hemp plants. CBD's impact on a molecular level is still being researched by scientists, but so far it has been shown to have a positive effect on many illnesses and to aid in sleep and relaxation.

WHAT IS THC?

THC, or tetrahydrocannabinol, is the chemical responsible for most of cannabis's psychoactive effects. THC is one of many compounds found in the resin secreted by glands of the cannabis plant and is highly sought-after. It stimulates cells in the brain to release dopamine, creating euphoria. It also interferes with how information is processed in the hippocampus, the area of the brain responsible for forming new memories. THC can induce hallucinations and alter thinking. On average, the effects last about two hours and kick in ten to thirty minutes after inhalation, or four to six hours when ingested (after kicking in after about thirty minutes).

WHAT ARE TERPENES?

Terpenes are the aromatic, or flavor, compounds found in all plants, fruits, and vegetables. In cannabis, terpenes are responsible for giving each strain its unique taste and smell—and experience for the user. When you purchase a particular strain, ask the dispensary for the strain certificate of analysis (COA), which will tell you the strain's chemical profile and enable you to look for it again, since strain names vary drastically by growers. You may also be able to look the strain up on the brand's website.

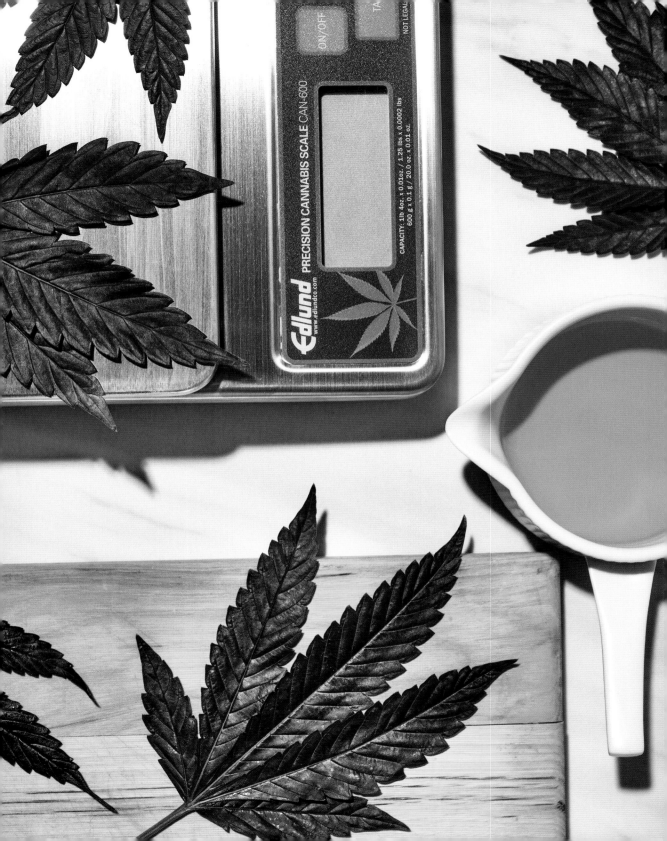

CHAPTER 2

COOKING WITH CANNABIS

Calculating Dosage

Consistent and reliable dosing is one of the most prized accomplishments of my company, The Herbal Chef. It's important to know how much cannabis you're taking in when you're baking edibles, just as it's important to know the ingredients of any food you're eating—or serving to friends and family. You must have an accurate and trustworthy digital scale. The simple equation below will enable you to determine the right amount of concentrate to weigh out to achieve precise dosing. If you follow it, you should get the right amount every time.

$$c = t/p$$

c equals the amount of concentrate

t equals the target amount of THC

p equals the decimal form of the percentage
of THC in your concentrate

Here are the rules we follow explained:

The value used for p **must be** in decimal form. This means that if we're working with a concentrate that is 75% THC, then $p = .75$. Similarly, if we're working with a concentrate that's 30% THC, our value for p will be .30, or simply .3.

Values for c and t **must be** measured in milligrams (mg). So if you are figuring out how much concentrate to use in your recipe to acquire 20 mg of THC in the dish from a concentrate that is 74% THC:

$$c = t/p = 20 \text{ mg}/.74 \approx 27.03 \text{ mg}$$

c is returned as a value in milligrams because we plugged in a milligram value for t.

SOME MORE EXAMPLES:

You want to add 10 mg of THC to a dish using a concentrate that is 75% THC. Begin by assigning the variables:

$$t = 10 \text{ mg}$$
$$p = .75$$
$$c = ?$$

Plug these values into the equation:

$$c = t/p = 10 \text{ mg}/.75 \approx 13.33 \text{ mg}$$

Therefore, you must add 13.33 mg of concentrate to the dish in order to add 10 mg of THC.

You're making a cannabis-infused confetti cake and want to add 3 milligrams (mg) of THC to the mixture using a concentrate that's 54% THC. How much concentrate must you use?

$$t = 3 \text{ mg}$$
$$p = .54$$
$$c = ?$$

Plugging these variables into our equation:

$c = t/p = 3 \text{ mg}/.54 \approx 5.56 \text{ mg}$

Therefore you must add 5.56 mg of concentrate to the cake batter in order to add 3 mg of THC. Notice our equation returned c in milligrams because our target amount of THC t was a value in milligrams.

How Are THC/CBD/Terpenes Derived from the Plants?

These compounds are derived from the plant in a few ways. The plant's flower is typically the source of extraction because it has the highest concentration of cannabinoids, terpenes, and flavonoids.

The leaves contain a negligible amount. Within the structure of the budding flower (hence the slang term *bud*) there are cellular molecular structures called *trichomes*. These are microscopic bubbles that hold all the abundant cannabinoids.

The process of extraction gently detaches the trichomes from the plant matter, which consists of fibers and other material. The fibers are used for clothing, bedding, housing material, and more, while the cannabinoids are used for ingestion, topical absorption, or inhalation. We'll start with a brief overview of the most well-known methods of consumption and extraction.

WAYS TO CONSUME

Smoking: This method only retains a small percentage of the compounds (5% to 20%) which in turn reduces the health advantages. It can cause damage in the lungs as well. Onset is immediate and lasts anywhere from one to two hours.

Vaporizing: This method retains a much higher percentage of compounds (45% to 70%) and can also be harmful to the lungs. The effect of this method can last anywhere from thirty minutes to one and a half hours. In this method, the cannabinoids are liberated through hot air and flow into the lungs.

Dabbing: This method retains nearly all of the compounds when used. Onset is immediate and usually lasts a much shorter amount of time, twenty to forty-five minutes. The quality is dependent on which extraction method is used.

Topicals: This method would be the next best way to introduce your fragile grandmother to the effects of the plant other than a very low dose edible. It doesn't impart a mental high; instead, it provides localized pain relief. This is crucial for anyone having physical pain or aches in a given body part, from their neck down to their feet!

WAYS TO EXTRACT

Ethanol Extraction: This method of extraction includes fractional distillation and pure ethanol with agitation. In other words, the ethanol breaks down the compounds from the plant matter, which then allows you to carefully extract the different cannabinoids by heating the solution to varying degrees. If you can heat the terpenes gently and uniformly, you can extract different terpenes at slightly varying degrees. Based on the temperature you are heating the solution to, the compounds in the ethanol will turn gaseous and you can trap them in another container.

Lipid Extraction: Here, you decarboxylate (or heat gently) the cannabis flower in an oven, then extract the lipid compounds into a fat. You can use oil, butter, or any other fat. Depending on the method, a typical extraction will only infuse 50% to 75% of the compounds in the plant. If you want to keep the terpenes intact, the extraction must be done in stages at corresponding temperatures. Most people who use this method aren't concerned with the terpenes staying intact as it's extremely tedious to retain them. The idea is that you grind up the cured cannabis, put it in a pot with any clarified or refined fat, then heat the pot on the stovetop on the lowest setting, or until it's 175°F. Let it steep for at least six hours to extract the maximum compounds.

Cold Water Extraction: Ice water, agitation, and fine sieves are employed to separate the compounds from the plant. Since the compounds are lipid soluble, they won't break down in the water. What this means is that you can grind the cured cannabis flower, put it in a fine mesh bag in an ice bath, and shake it vigorously until the trichomes separate from the plant matter that's in the bag. The strainers used are different sizes to catch different particles.

Butane Extraction: There's a lot of room for error here. After supercooling the plant matter and flushing it through a tube, you must gently warm the extracted product to evaporate the butane so you're left with just the compounds. This has a high risk of leaving in some butane, which is toxic for the body to ingest. Purging the butane from the final product is of the utmost importance for this method.

CO_2 Extraction: This is a flushing method as well, but CO_2 is less harmful to the body than butane and is more easily purged from the final product. The extraction is created by forcing pressurized carbon dioxide into a vessel with biomass and then separating the waxes, terpenes, and cannabinoids from the plant fibers and gas used for the extraction.

Best Practices for Enjoying Cannabis

Cannabis is like a lover. Take your time getting to know the intricacies of the experience, move slowly, and you will develop a lasting relationship with the plant.

Cannabis should never, *never* be forced upon anyone who is not consenting. In other words, you can never serve a cannabis-infused dessert to someone unless that person is completely aware of what is in the dish. Cannabis is a wonderful accent to an overall healthy lifestyle, but it is just a *part* of a lifestyle. If it is the only thing in your life that's adding value, or if you find yourself relying on it too much to feel good, then you must take stock: Are you too dependent on it? Are there areas of your life that you need to assess? Cannabis enhances life, but it should not be used to make life good or to lessen the glare of things that aren't great.

It is natural to have a relationship that ebbs and flows. You may use cannabis with more frequency at certain times and less at others, or you may need to take a break from it altogether. Everyone finds their own balance and understanding of how cannabis adds to their life.

Responsible Dosing: It takes time to develop an understanding of how much THC is the right amount for you. Everyone metabolizes cannabis differently: there is no "one size fits all" approach. So, start slowly and conservatively. Responsible dosing is understanding how much cannabis is in your dish and how it affects you. And, if you're serving it to others, it is your essential responsibility to convey the correct milligrams in the product so that others can make an informed decision about whether to eat it and how much to eat based on how they respond to cannabis. This is vital.

Alcohol & THC: Simply put, alcohol is a catalyst for the metabolism of the psychoactive component of cannabis, THC. That means if you decide to consume both alcohol and edibles, the alcohol will trigger a faster and stronger effect of the edibles than you may be anticipating. Again, take it slow. Find your balance. You can always have another drink, but you can't undo what you've eaten, so make sure to exercise caution when having cannabis-infused desserts with alcohol.

How to Use CBD

Our endocannabinoid system does not always receive the amounts of naturally produced cannabidiol it needs. If you can include it in your meals or baked goods through an oil, this would be my preferred method for supplementation, as it's highly bioavailable through ingestion. Another method would be to take it sublingually (under the tongue) via an oil or tincture. I can't help it if my favorite way to take my CBD is with chocolate ganache.

How to Use Terpenes

Terpenes are the aromatic, flavor, and color profile of a given strain of cannabis. Terpenes are present in the oils of just about all botanicals, vegetables, and fruits. With increasing research into the field of cannabis pharmacology, there are many studies depicting the importance of terpenes and how they provide much more than aroma and flavor. They can be responsible for helping limit bacterial growth or even stopping it completely in what's referred to as an "entourage effect" with the other compounds found in cannabis. In some clinical trials, it's been shown that a combination of CBD, THC, and terpenes can be responsible for improving cognitive function and memory in patients.[3] On page 144 you can find a reputable source to order terpenes to use in cooking, drinks, or even your diffuser. Just a drop in any of the above will do. We use a ratio of .01% of the total weight of something when adding terpenes.

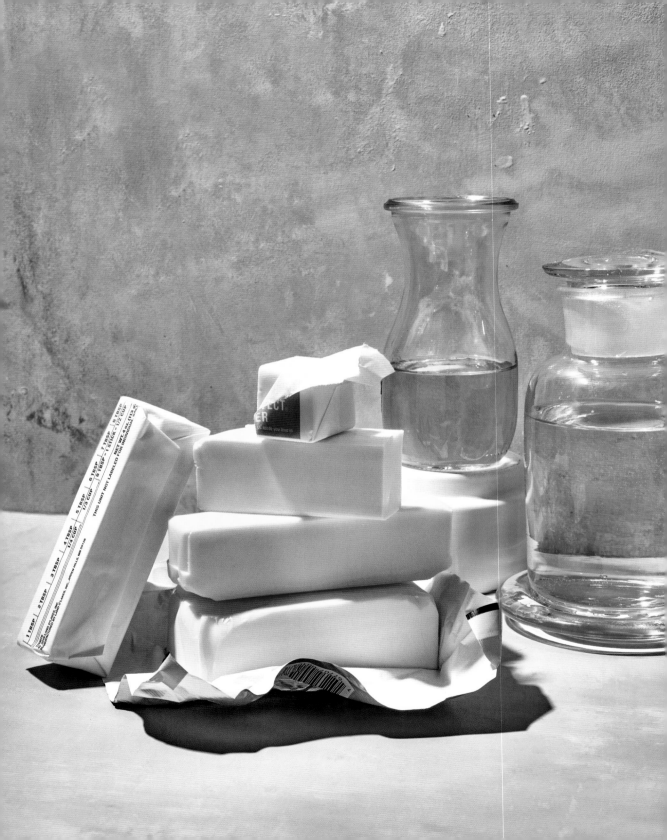

CHAPTER 3

Infusions

If you can't find cannabis tinctures, concentrates, or ready-made infusions, it's easy to make basic ones that will allow you to bake anything.

Before we get into it, I have to caution you: there's absolutely no way of *definitively* knowing what the dosage of these infusions are unless you know the starting potency of the flower you're using and you're sure you'll get 100 percent yield of all the cannabinoids from the plant into your infusion. That doesn't mean you can't make your own and experiment little by little to see what works for you! Remember to start out with just a little bit, then see how you feel after two hours before trying more. That means try out a teaspoon in a recipe and monitor your high; if you feel like you could go for more, increase the dosage slowly until you get into a comfortable zone. You can always add more, but you can't take it away!

When baking with infusions, you can add them to the recipe when the oil or the butter is being added. Add tinctures where the liquid is used. In savory recipes, add the infusion toward the end of the cooking process to be sure you aren't overheating the infusion and mitigating its potency. In the recipes that follow, the ingredient printed in green indicates where to add the cannabis. For instance, if you are making a tomato tart with caramelized onion on the bottom with fresh tomatoes and herbs on the top, add the infusion to the dressing that will go on top of the tomatoes, not in the cooking process of the onions, because the heat can degrade the potency.

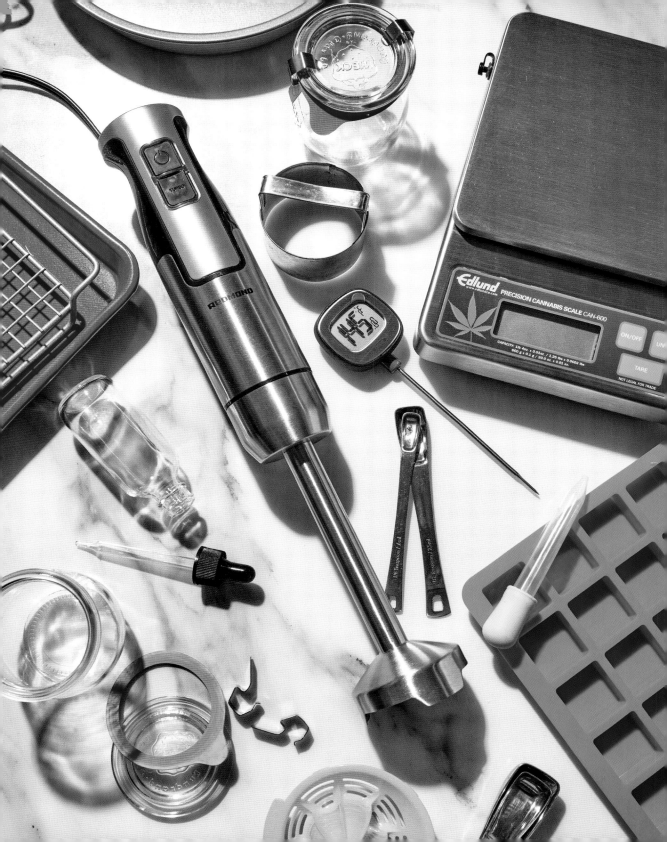

Easy-to-Find Equipment for Making Cannabis-Infused Treats

Herb grinder

Food scale

Cheesecloth

Rubber bands

Parchment paper

Plastic wrap

Glass airtight storage jars, such as Ball or Weck

Candy thermometer

Chef's thermometer

Slow cooker

Food processor

Stand mixer

Blender or immersion blender

Cast-iron skillet or Dutch oven

Ice cream maker

Carbonation device

Rimmed sheet pans (9 × 13 inch, 8 × 8 inch)

Baking dishes (8 × 8 inch, 9 × 13 inch)

Tart pans (10 inch)

Cake pans (9 inch)

Pie pans (9 inch)

Six-ounce ramekins

Large, heavy pot

Bowls (small, medium, and large)

Sauté pans

Sauce pans (small, medium, and large)

Double boiler or heatproof bowl

Pastry bag or sturdy zip-top bag

Ladle

Sifter

Whisk

Spatula

Wooden spoon

Chocolate molds

Nonstick Silpat

Large cookie scoop

Fine mesh strainer

Tea towel

Pie weights

Cookie stamp/cookie press/cookie cutter

Slotted spoon

Offset spatula/knife

Rubber spatula

Culinary torch

Wire rack/cake rack

Springform pan (9 inch)

Cake tester or toothpicks

Aluminum foil

Pastry cutter

Tongs

Pastry brush

Oil Infusion

YIELD: **1 CUP**

3.5 grams of your favorite cannabis (or you can use "already-vaporized bud" [AVB])

1 cup coconut, avocado, or other oil

1. Preheat the oven to 350°F. Line a rimmed sheet pan with parchment paper.

2. Weigh and grind the cannabis to a small grind; it should be light and fluffy. Spread it in an even layer on the prepared sheet pan. Bake for 30 minutes, or until the cannabis is just past golden brown. There will be a vaporized cannabis aroma coming from the oven. Remove the sheet pan from the oven and set aside to cool.

3. Pour the oil into a small saucepan over low heat. Once the oil reaches 165°F to 175°F, remove it from the heat and add the decarboxylated (baked) cannabis to the saucepan. Let it sit for at least 12 hours at room temperature, stirring it every few hours and bringing it back up to 165°F to 175°F over low heat when it drops below 100°F. Alternatively, you can do this in a slow cooker on the lowest setting.

4. With a cheesecloth, make a square approximately double the size of the opening of an 8 oz glass jar. Using a rubber band, secure the cheesecloth around the mouth of the jar. Strain the oil through the cheesecloth into the jar. Let the oil cool completely before placing the lid on the jar. Clearly label the jar with the strain, amount of cannabis used, and amount of oil, and store it in a cool, dry place.

RECIPE TIP: Increasing the cook time won't hurt your end product; however, it's very important that the temperature stays between 165°F and 175°F. Always be monitoring!

Butter Infusion

YIELD: **1 CUP**

4 cups unsalted butter (I like organic butter made with milk from grass-fed cows) or prepared ghee

3.5 grams of your favorite cannabis (or you can use AVB)

1. Preheat the oven to 350˚F. Line a rimmed sheet pan with parchment paper.

2. Place the butter in a medium saucepan over medium-low heat and cook until it is completely melted.

3. Weigh and grind the cannabis to a small grind; it should be light and fluffy. Spread it in an even layer on the prepared sheet pan. Bake for 30 minutes, or until the cannabis is just past golden brown. There will be a vaporized cannabis aroma coming from the oven. Remove the sheet pan from the oven and set aside to cool.

4. Meanwhile, once the butter is melted, using a spoon, skim the white milk solids from the top. Keep skimming until you have a clarified butter, also known as ghee. Pour the ghee into a bowl and set aside.

5. Wipe out the pot with a paper towel to make sure that none of the particles remain. Return 1 cup of the ghee to the saucepan and gently warm over low heat until a thermometer reads 165˚F to 175˚F. Let it cook for 2 to 3 hours. Once the butter is stabilized, remove it from the heat, add the decarboxylated (baked) cannabis, and let it steep for 12 hours, stirring it every once in a while.

6. With a cheesecloth, make a square approximately double the size of the opening of an 8 oz glass jar. Using a rubber band, secure the cheesecloth around the mouth of the jar. Strain the butter through the cheesecloth and into the jar. Let the clarified butter cool completely before placing the lid on the jar. Clearly label the jar with the strain, amount of cannabis used, and amount of butter, and store it in the refrigerator or freezer. It will keep in the refrigerator for 3 months and in the freezer for a year, so feel free to make a big batch ahead of time.

Tincture

YIELD: **1 CUP**

3.5 grams of your favorite cannabis (or you can use AVB)

1 cup any high-proof alcohol (I prefer a clear alcohol 70 proof or above)

1. Preheat the oven to 350°F. Line a rimmed sheet pan with parchment paper.

2. Weigh and grind the cannabis to a small grind; it should be light and fluffy. Spread it in an even layer on the prepared sheet pan. Bake for 30 minutes, or until the cannabis is just past golden brown. There will be a vaporized cannabis aroma coming from the oven. Remove the sheet pan from the oven and set aside to cool.

3. Pour the alcohol into an 8 oz glass jar and add the decarboxylated (baked) cannabis. Secure the lid and swirl the alcohol and cannabis so that the cannabis becomes incorporated into the liquid.

4. Vigorously shake the jar a few times daily for 2 weeks.

5. With a cheesecloth, make a square approximately double the size of the opening of the jar. Using a rubber band, secure the cheesecloth around the mouth of the jar. Pour the cannabis-alcohol mixture through the cheesecloth to strain it. Using a funnel, pour the liquid into a dropper bottle clearly labeled with the strain, amount of cannabis used, and amount of tincture, and store in a cool, dry place. It will be good for up to one year.

You've made it! Welcome to the holy land of cannabis-infused sweet treats.

Before you read on, please know you can create your own dosage in each recipe. If you have a lab-tested extract, you can use the algorithm on page 24 to get the exact dosage you're looking for. If you only have your at-home infusion, then test it out a teaspoon at a time so you can find your tolerance level.

When you are first making a recipe, I highly recommend starting with a low dose. If it's not enough the first time, you can always go higher the second time around. You will add the infused butter, oil, or tincture to the recipe where the fat is added. Just replace the amount of regular fat with the amount of infusion you're using, and you'll be ready to go. For example, if the recipe calls for 300 grams of butter and you're adding 8 grams of cannabis butter, then you add 292 grams of regular butter with the 8 grams of infused butter to complete the recipe. Four grams roughly equals one teaspoon. Remember to do the math!

In addition, all of these recipes have been tested to be made gluten free by adding in a cup-for-cup gluten-free flour replacement. You can also make them dairy free by using nondairy alternatives.

Last note, please make sure to label your treats so they don't get confused with their cannabis-less counterparts!

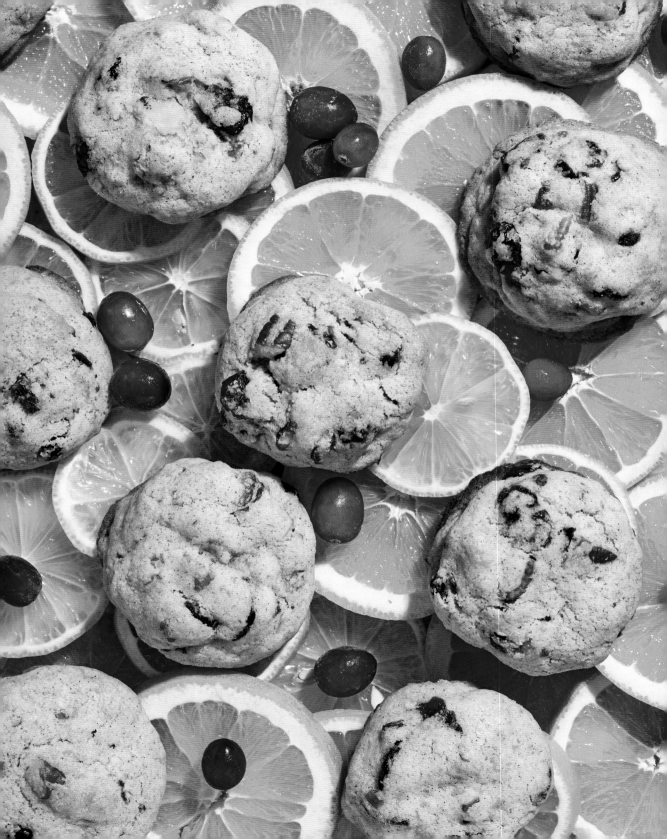

CHAPTER 4

COOKIES, BROWNIES & BARS

Brown Butter Salted Chocolate Chip Cookies

YIELD: 24 COOKIES

Oh look, another chocolate chip cookie recipe. But this, *this* is *the* chocolate chip cookie recipe you need. The brown butter combined with the rich dark chocolate and walnuts create a thing of true beauty and deliciousness. I use cream of tartar in many of my baked goods because I think it gives cookies and bars a superior texture of airiness. These cookies are similar to the wildly popular Levain cookie. But dare I say better? Share them and enjoy.

1 cup (2 sticks) unsalted butter (226 grams)

2½ cups all-purpose flour (300 grams)

1 teaspoon baking soda (4 grams)

¾ teaspoon kosher salt (4 grams)

½ teaspoon cream of tartar (1.6 grams)

¾ cup light brown sugar (193 grams)

⅔ cup granulated sugar (134 grams)

1 large egg, at room temperature (50 grams)

1 large egg yolk, at room temperature (18 grams)

1 tablespoon pure vanilla extract (12 grams)

2 cups dark chocolate chips (342 grams)

¾ cup walnuts, toasted and chopped (100 grams)

Flaky salt, for garnish

1. In a medium sauté pan over medium heat, melt butter until it begins to foam. Swirl the butter in the pan to prevent it from burning, and allow it to cook until foaming stops, brown bits form on the bottom of the pan, and it smells nutty, 5 to 7 minutes. Remove from heat. Pour the butter into the bowl of a stand mixer fitted with the paddle attachment and let it cool at room temperature for 2 hours, or until solid but still soft.

2. Into a medium bowl, sift together the flour, baking soda, salt, and cream of tartar, then whisk until well combined. Set aside.

3. Add the brown sugar and granulated sugar to the room-temperature butter and cream together on medium speed until light and fluffy, 3 to 4 minutes. Add the whole egg and mix until incorporated. Then add egg yolk and mix until well combined.

4. Scrape down the sides of the bowl, then add the vanilla and mix at medium speed for 1 minute.

5. Add the flour mixture to the butter and mix on low just until a few streaks of flour remain. Remove the bowl from the stand mixer and fold in the chocolate chips and walnuts by hand until evenly dispersed. Cover dough with plastic wrap and refrigerate overnight.

6. When ready to bake, line two rimmed baking sheets with parchment paper and preheat the oven to 375°F. Scoop the cookie dough using a large (size 16) cookie scoop (dough balls should be about 60 grams each) and place about 6 on each prepared baking sheet, making sure to leave 3 to 4 inches for the cookies to spread.

7. Sprinkle with flaky salt to taste and bake for 9 minutes, or until golden brown. The center of the cookies will be very soft; let them firm up on the baking sheet for 2 minutes after removing them from the oven, then move them to a wire rack to cool completely. Repeat with remaining dough.

TIP: You can make the brown butter in step one ahead of time and refrigerate it. Just make sure that it comes to room temperature before creaming it with the sugars. You can also store brown butter in the freezer for up to 9 months.

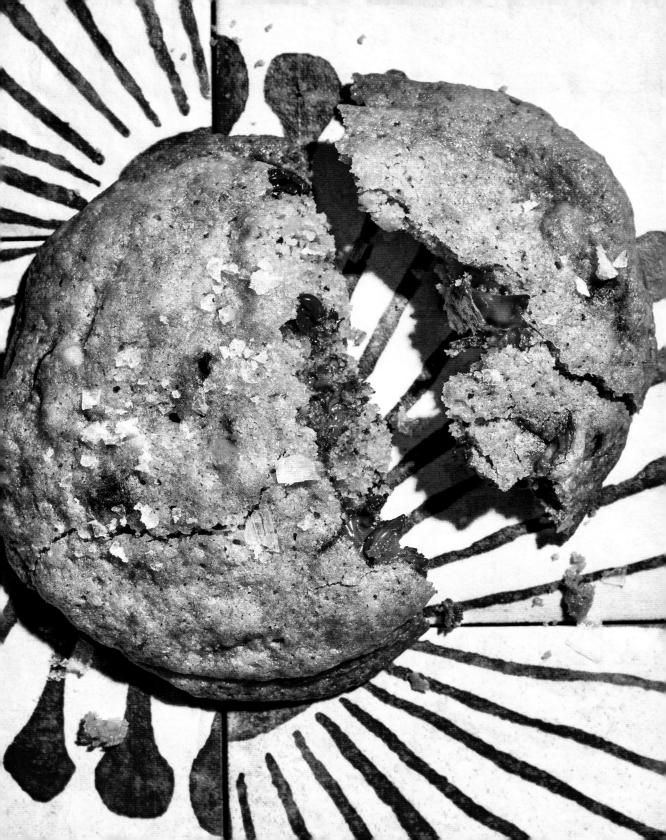

Banana Cream Pie Cookies

YIELD: 36 COOKIES

Move over banana bread, banana cream pie cookies are the way to use up those shabby-looking bananas. The recipe for the banana pudding used here will yield more than you need for these cookies, but the leftovers are great for dipping strawberries, apples, bananas, or any other sturdy fruit. It's also great as a morning oatmeal topper.

3½ cups all-purpose flour (452 grams)

1½ teaspoons baking soda (6 grams)

¾ teaspoon kosher salt (4 grams)

1 cup (2 sticks) unsalted butter, at room temperature (224 grams)

1 cup granulated sugar (200 grams)

1 cup packed brown sugar (192 grams)

1½ cups banana pudding (380 grams), recipe follows

2 large eggs (100 grams)

1½ teaspoons vanilla extract (6 grams)

1½ cups white chocolate chips (257 grams)

5 graham cracker sheets, coarsely broken into chunks (77 grams)

TIP: You can make this dough a day ahead and store it in the refrigerator for up to 3 days before baking.

1. Into a medium bowl, sift together the flour, baking soda, and salt, then whisk until well combined. Set aside.

2. In the bowl of a stand mixer fitted with the paddle attachment, cream the butter, granulated sugar, and brown sugar on high speed until pale and fluffy, about 4 minutes.

3. Add the banana pudding, eggs, and vanilla to the butter mixture and beat on medium speed until fully incorporated, about 1 minute. Slowly add the flour mixture and beat until no streaks of flour remain. Add the white chocolate chips and crushed graham crackers, mixing until just combined. Cover the dough with plastic wrap and refrigerate for at least 2 hours.

4. When ready to bake, preheat the oven to 350°F and line two rimmed baking sheets with parchment paper. Scoop dough into 2½-tablespoon portions (50 grams). Place the dough on the prepared baking sheets 2 inches apart, and bake 9 to 11 minutes, or until golden brown. Let the cookies sit for 5 minutes on the baking sheets, then transfer them to a wire rack and let cool completely.

Banana Pudding

4 very overripe bananas (575 grams)

1 (¼-ounce) packet gelatin powder (7 grams)

½ cup whole or plant-based milk (120 grams)

1. In a medium bowl, mash the bananas, then sprinkle the gelatin evenly on top.

2. In a small saucepan over medium heat, gently warm the milk for about 2 minutes. Do not let it boil.

3. Transfer the bananas and geletin to a blender and pour in the warm milk. Blend on high. Alternatively, you can do this in a large mixing bowl using an immersion blender.

4. Strain the mixture through a fine mesh strainer set over a medium bowl. Cover with plastic wrap and let chill in the refrigerator for at least 2 hours or up to overnight.

OG Sugar Cookies

In the lineup of classic cookies, I had to throw in the OG sugar cookie. I love these for their simplicity. There's nothing here but the cookie and you. Namaste.

3⅔ cups all-purpose flour (458 grams)

1½ teaspoons baking powder (6 grams)

2 teaspoons kosher salt (12 grams)

1½ cups (3 sticks) unsalted butter, at room temperature (339 grams)

1⅓ cups granulated sugar, plus more for rolling (336 grams)

2 large eggs, at room temperature (100 grams)

1 tablespoon pure vanilla extract (12 grams)

1. Into a medium bowl, sift together the flour, baking powder, and salt, then whisk until well combined. Set aside.

2. In the bowl of a stand mixer fitted with the paddle attachment, add the butter and sugar and cream together on medium speed until light and fluffy, 3 to 4 minutes.

3. Scrape down the sides of the bowl, then add the eggs one at a time, mixing on medium speed until each egg is fully incorporated. Scrape down the sides of the bowl again, then add the vanilla and mix until combined.

4. Add the flour mixture to the butter and sugar mixture, and mix until just fully incorporated and no streaks of flour remain. Cover the dough with plastic wrap and refrigerate for at least 12 hours.

5. When ready to bake, preheat the oven to 350°F and line two rimmed baking sheets with parchment paper.

6. Using a large cookie scoop, scoop the dough into 2 tablespoon–size balls (about 50 grams each). Roll each dough ball in granulated sugar, then place the cookies on the prepared baking sheets, leaving 3 inches in between each cookie.

7. Bake for 9 to 11 minutes, rotating the baking sheets front to back and top to bottom halfway through baking time. Remove the cookies from the oven and let them sit on the baking sheets for 1 minute before transferring to a wire rack to cool completely. Repeat with the remaining dough.

Tahini Cookies

YIELD: 24 COOKIES

As a Middle Eastern man, I wanted to include a few family recipes. While most kids use peanut butter from the pantry when they feel like baking something sweet, I would reach for tahini paste, which was always in my *jiddeh*'s pantry. To this day, I always have it on hand. This dough works best with an overnight chill, so it's a perfect make-ahead recipe, too. Halvah is available at most supermarkets, but if you can't find it, there are many good brands available online.

3 cups all-purpose flour (375 grams)

2 teaspoons baking soda (8 grams)

1 teaspoon baking powder (4 grams)

¾ teaspoon kosher salt (3 grams)

1 cup (2 sticks) unsalted butter, at room temperature (224 grams)

1 cup plus 2 tablespoons granulated sugar (225 grams)

1 cup packed dark brown sugar (212 grams)

1 cup tahini paste (263 grams)

2 large eggs (100 grams)

1 cup crumbled halvah (sesame confection) (140 grams)

¼ cup black sesame seeds (35 grams)

1. Into a medium bowl, sift together the flour, baking soda, baking powder, and salt, then whisk until well combined. Set aside.

2. In the bowl of a stand mixer fitted with the paddle attachment, add the butter, granulated sugar, and brown sugar and cream together on medium speed until pale and fluffy, 3 to 4 minutes. Add the tahini and mix until fully combined.

3. Scrape down the sides of the bowl, then add the eggs one at a time, mixing on medium speed until each egg is fully incorporated, 2 to 3 minutes.

4. Gradually add the flour mixture to the bowl of the stand mixer and mix on low speed until the flour has been incorporated, taking care not to overmix. Add the halvah and sesame seeds and mix on low speed until just incorporated. Scrape the dough into a medium bowl. Cover the dough with plastic wrap and refrigerate for at least 2 hours or up to overnight.

5. When ready to bake, preheat the oven to 375°F and line two rimmed baking sheets with parchment paper. Using a large cookie scoop, scoop the dough into 2 tablespoon–size balls (about 50 grams each) and place them 2 inches apart on the prepared baking sheets.

6. Bake for 10 to 12 minutes, or until golden brown. The cookies will be soft, so do not overbake. Remove the cookies from the oven and let them sit on the baking sheets for 1 to 2 minutes before transferring to a wire rack to cool completely.

TIP: The dough, covered in plastic wrap, will keep in the refrigerator for up to 3 days. You can bake just a few cookies at a time for spur-of-the-moment freshly baked treats.

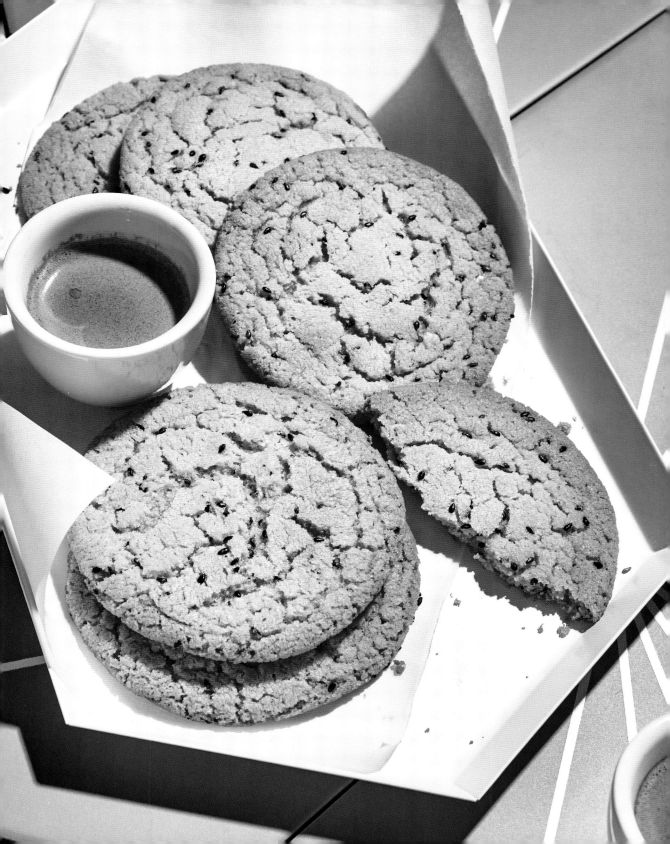

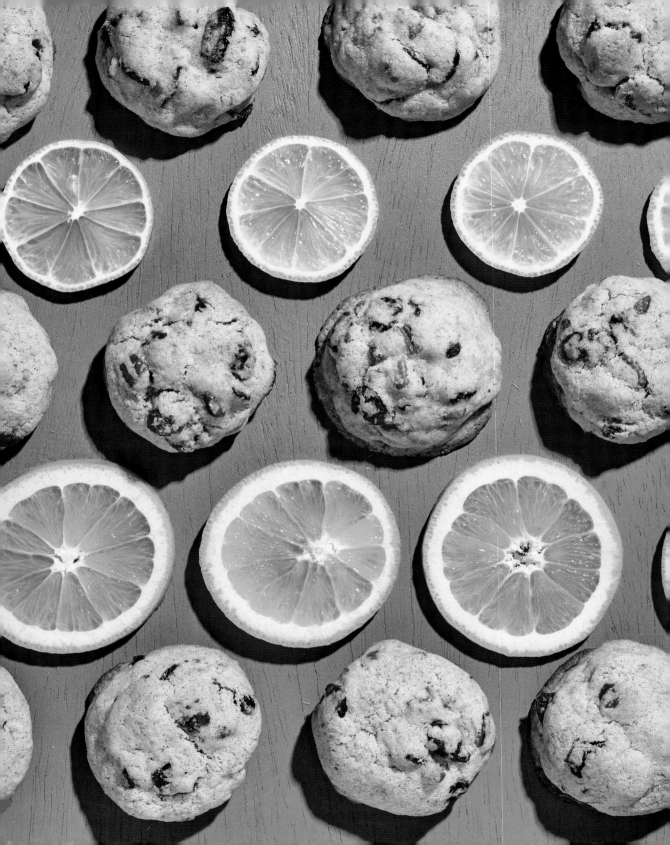

Citrus-Cranberry Cookies

YIELD: 16 COOKIES

I'm all about diversity of flavor, and these cookies are probably not what you are used to finding in your cookie jar! I'm big on chocolate, but chocolate cookies can be rich and heavy, so I wanted to include something that was on the lighter side, with bright citrus notes complemented by the aromatic spices that are frequently used in Middle Eastern recipes. The cranberries pair well with the fluffy cookie and the crunch of the pecans. This will be your new crowd favorite.

¾ cup granulated sugar (150 grams)

1 tablespoon (6 grams) fresh orange zest, from about 2 medium oranges

½ tablespoon (3 grams) fresh lemon zest, from ½ medium lemon

1¾ cups all-purpose flour (219 grams)

¾ teaspoon baking powder (about 3 grams)

1 teaspoon ground allspice (about 2 grams)

Pinch of ground anise

1 teaspoon kosher salt (6 grams)

½ cup plus 4 tablespoons unsalted butter, at room temperature (168 grams)

1 large egg, at room temperature (50 grams)

¾ teaspoon pure vanilla extract (3 grams)

1 cup sweetened dried cranberries (135 grams)

¾ cup shelled pecans, chopped (92 grams)

1. In a medium bowl, add the sugar, orange zest, and lemon zest. Work the zest into the sugar with your fingers to release the citrus oils. Set aside.

2. Into a separate medium bowl, sift together the flour, baking powder, allspice, anise, and salt, then whisk until well combined. Set aside.

3. In the bowl of a stand mixer fitted with the paddle attachment, combine the butter and citrus sugar and cream on medium speed until light and fluffy, 3 to 4 minutes.

4. Scrape down the sides of the bowl with a spatula, then add the egg and vanilla and mix on medium speed for 2 to 3 minutes, or until well combined.

5. Gradually add the flour mixture to the butter and sugar mixture and mix just until no streaks of flour remain. Add the cranberries and pecans and mix on low speed until well combined. Cover the dough with plastic wrap and refrigerate for at least 3 hours.

6. When ready to bake, preheat the oven to 375°F and line two rimmed baking sheets with parchment paper.

7. Using a large cookie scoop, scoop the dough into 2 tablespoon–size balls (about 50 grams each). Place the cookies on the prepared baking sheets, leaving 3 inches in between each cookie.

8. Bake for 10 to 12 minutes, rotating the baking sheets front to back and top to bottom halfway through baking time. Remove the cookies from the oven and allow them to sit on the baking sheets for 1 minute, then transfer them to a wire rack to cool completely. Repeat with remaining dough.

Double Chocolate Cookies

YIELD: **24 COOKIES**

If you looked up this double chocolate cookie in the dictionary, I'm pretty sure it would be defined as *heavenly*. This recipe is straight from my heart, and one of my true favorites because it is filled with ooey, gooey, chocolaty goodness. Enjoy your piece of heaven!

2¾ cups all-purpose flour (344 grams)

½ cup Dutch-processed cocoa powder (57 grams)

1 teaspoon baking powder (4 grams)

¾ teaspoon kosher salt (4 grams)

½ teaspoon cream of tartar (1.6 grams)

1 cup (2 sticks) unsalted butter, at room temperature (224 grams)

⅔ cup granulated sugar (132 grams)

¾ cup plus 1 tablespoon packed dark brown sugar (193 grams)

1 large egg, at room temperature (50 grams)

1 large egg yolk, at room temperature (18 grams)

1 tablespoon pure vanilla extract (12 grams)

2 cups dark chocolate chunks (342 grams)

Flaky salt, to finish

1. Into a medium bowl, sift together the flour, cocoa powder, baking powder, salt, and cream of tartar, then whisk until well combined. Set aside.

2. In the bowl of a stand mixer fitted with the paddle attachment, add the butter, granulated sugar, and brown sugar and cream together on medium speed until pale and fluffy, 3 to 4 minutes. Add the egg and egg yolk, one at a time, then add the vanilla. Mix thoroughly until fully incorporated.

3. Add the flour mixture to the bowl of the stand mixer and mix on low speed just until no streaks of flour remain, 1 minute.

4. Fold the chocolate chunks into the batter with a spatula. Cover the dough with plastic wrap and refrigerate for at least 4 hours.

5. When ready to bake, preheat the oven to 350°F and line two rimmed baking sheets with parchment paper. Using a large cookie scoop, scoop the dough into 2 tablespoon–size balls (about 57 grams each) and place them about 3 inches apart on the prepared baking sheets.

6. Bake for 9 to 11 minutes, rotating the baking sheets front to back and top to bottom halfway through baking time. Remove the cookies from the oven and allow them to sit on the baking sheets for 1 minute, then transfer to a wire rack. Sprinkle each warm cookie with flaky salt, then leave to cool completely.

7. Repeat the baking process with the remaining cookie dough.

Dulce de Leche Coconut Blondies

YIELD: **16 BLONDIES**

I feel like every blondie I see out there is the same thing over and over, with the caramel brittle and chocolate chips, so I decided to change all that with these decadent dulce de leche–based blondies. They are well balanced and super rich and can compete with even the best brownies (i.e., my space brownies!!).

1 cup canned coconut cream, at room temperature (189 grams)

⅓ cup prepared dulce de leche, at room temperature (113 grams)

3 tablespoons unsalted butter, softened (42 grams)

3 large eggs, at room temperature (150 grams)

1 cup coconut sugar (162 grams)

½ tablespoon pure vanilla extract (6 grams)

1¾ cups all-purpose flour (219 grams)

1¾ teaspoons baking powder (7 grams)

1 teaspoon kosher salt (6 grams)

1¾ cups white chocolate chips (276 grams)

1. Preheat the oven to 350°F and line an 8 × 8-inch baking dish with parchment paper, leaving a little bit hanging over the sides.

2. In a large bowl, whisk the coconut cream, dulce de leche, and butter until well combined. Set aside.

3. In a medium bowl, whisk the eggs and coconut sugar until thick, fluffy, and smooth, about 2 minutes. Add the vanilla and whisk again until fully incorporated, then transfer to the bowl with the coconut cream mixture and whisk until combined.

4. In a medium bowl, add the flour, baking powder, and salt and whisk to break up any lumps. Add the dry ingredients to the wet ingredients, folding in the flour mixture until no streaks of flour remain.

5. Scrape the batter into the prepared baking dish, spreading it into an even layer with an offset spatula. Sprinkle the white chocolate chips on top and bake for 20 to 25 minutes, or until the blondies have evenly risen and the center is dry to the touch.

6. Cool completely on a wire rack, then cut the blondies into 16 equal-size bars (68 grams each).

Space Brownies

When I first started college, the only edibles I could find were cereal treats and brownies. These weren't just any edibles. These were possibly the strongest edibles in California, which, if you were a novice, would have you packing your bags and taking flight. I've worked over the years to develop a brownie that was everything I really wanted in a chocolate morsel. The secret is to stir the eggs, rather than beat them. That's what makes these brownies super fudgy.

1 cup (2 sticks) unsalted butter, at room temperature (224 grams), plus more for the pan

1 (12-ounce) bag semisweet chocolate chips (340 grams), divided

½ cup Dutch-processed cocoa powder (57 grams)

3 large eggs, at room temperature (150 grams)

1⅔ cups granulated sugar (333 grams)

½ tablespoon pure vanilla extract (6 grams)

1¾ cups all-purpose flour (219 grams), plus more for the pan

2 teaspoons baking powder (8 grams)

1 teaspoon kosher salt (6 grams)

1. Preheat the oven to 350°F. Line a rimmed 8 × 12-inch baking dish with parchment paper, then butter and flour the entire surface.

2. In a double boiler, or in a large heatproof bowl set over a medium saucepan of simmering water (taking care not to let the bowl touch the water), add the butter, 4 ounces (½ cup) of chocolate chips, and the cocoa powder to the bowl and cook, stirring constantly, until smooth, 5 to 7 minutes. Remove from heat and allow it to cool slightly.

3. In a large bowl, *stir* together the eggs, sugar, and vanilla; do not beat. Stir the warm chocolate mixture into the egg mixture and allow to cool to room temperature.

4. In a medium bowl, fold the flour, baking powder, salt, and remaining 8 ounces (1 cup) chocolate chips together. Add to the cooled chocolate mixture and fold until just combined and no streaks of flour remain.

5. Scrape the batter into the prepared baking dish and bake for 20 to 25 minutes, or until a toothpick inserted into the center comes out clean. Do not overbake. Allow the brownies to cool completely, then refrigerate them for at least 2 hours before cutting into 24 equal-size brownies.

TIP: Serve with a scoop of vanilla ice cream and some chocolate fudge drizzle to really make this sing!

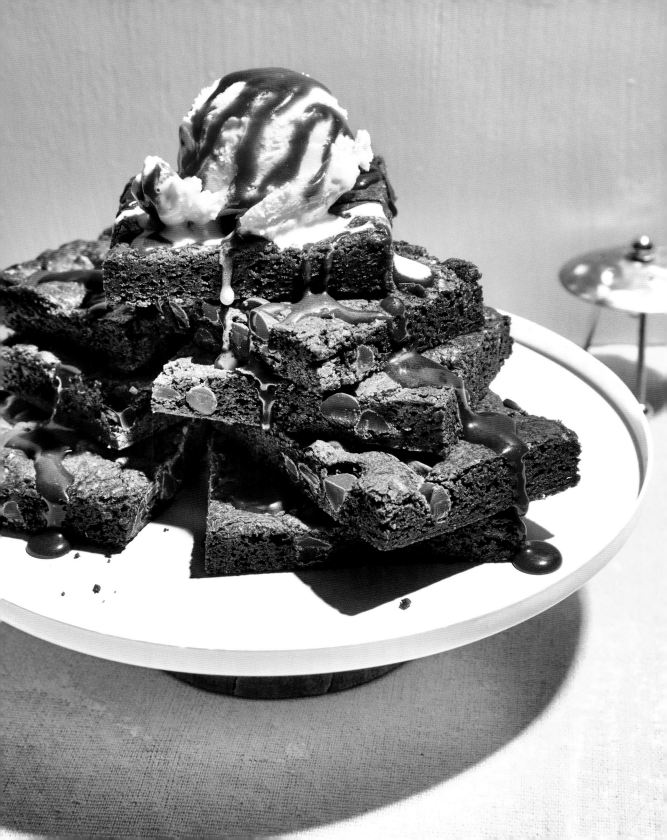

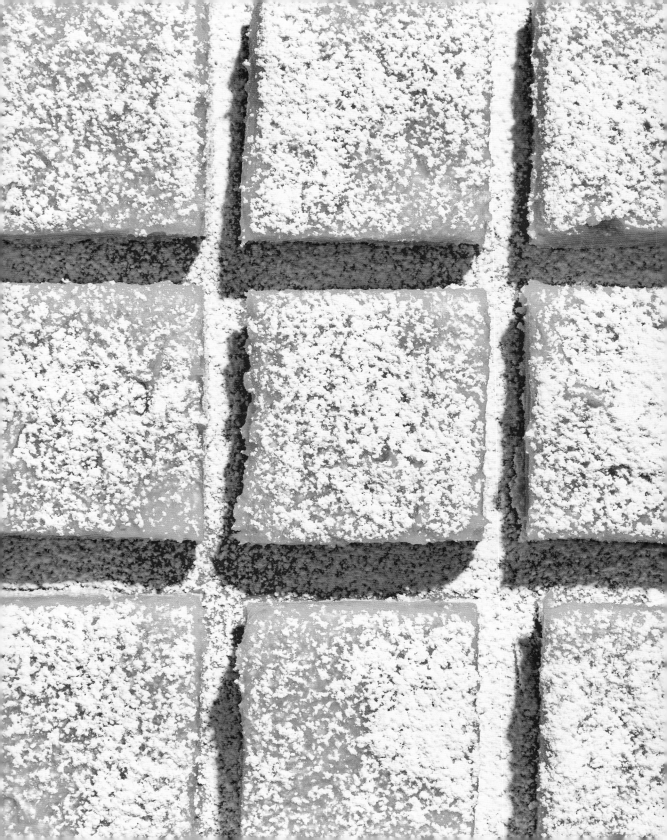

Lemon Bars

YIELD: **16 BARS**

I absolutely love a good lemon bar. Shortbread plus a gooey, zingy, creamy filling is something we can all gush over. This recipe is citrus versatile. By swapping a third of the lemon juice for fresh grapefruit, lime, or blood orange juice, you can customize these bars to become your own personal favorite!

FOR THE PASTRY CRUST

2½ cups all-purpose flour (312 grams)

2 tablespoons granulated sugar (25 grams)

2 teaspoons kosher salt (8 grams)

1 cup plus 4 tablespoons (2½ sticks) unsalted butter, chilled and cut into cubes (280 grams)

¼ cup cold water (50 grams)

FOR THE LEMON CURD

1½ cups granulated sugar (300 grams)

9 large egg yolks (162 grams)

1¼ cups strained, freshly squeezed lemon juice (from about 9 large lemons), or any citrus juice (300 grams)

½ cup (1 stick) plus 3 tablespoons unsalted butter (154 grams)

2 tablespoons fresh lemon zest (from about 4 large lemons) (15 grams)

½ teaspoon almond extract (2 grams)

¾ cup all-purpose flour (100 grams)

Confectioners' sugar, for garnish

1. **Make the pastry crust:** In a large bowl, add the flour, sugar, and salt and whisk until combined. Add the cold butter to the bowl. Using your fingers or a pastry cutter, work the butter into the flour until pea-size clumps form and the mixture becomes crumbly. Add the cold water, kneading by hand until a smooth dough forms. Cover the dough and let it rest in the refrigerator for 10 minutes. The dough can be made a day ahead as well.

2. Meanwhile, preheat the oven to 350°F and line a 9 × 13-inch baking dish with parchment paper. Remove the pastry crust from the refrigerator and press it into the bottom of the prepared pan. Bake the crust for 15 to 20 minutes, or until golden brown. Remove from the oven and set it aside to cool while you make the lemon curd.

3. **Make the lemon curd:** In a medium bowl, whisk the sugar and egg yolks together by hand until light and creamy, about 2 minutes. Set aside.

4. In a heavy-bottomed medium saucepan over medium heat, add the lemon juice, butter, lemon zest, and almond extract. Stir constantly for 3 minutes to avoid any burning on the bottom of the pan. Add the sugar and egg yolk mixture to the saucepan and continue to cook, mixing constantly, for 1 minute more. Add the flour and whisk until fully incorporated. Cook, whisking constantly, for 3 to 5 minutes or until the curd starts to thicken and coats the back of a spoon. Remove from heat. The curd will continue to thicken as it cools.

5. With a rubber spatula or an offset spatula, spread the lemon curd on top of the cooled tart shell. Chill for at least 3 hours in the refrigerator before cutting into 16 equal-size bars. Dust with confectioners' sugar and serve.

S'mores Bars

Camping is one of my all-time favorite activities. Out in nature I am invigorated, but I also feel a tremendous sense of calm at the same time. But the best part of camping? Probably the s'mores! When it comes to making s'mores, I'm quite particular. The chocolate needs to be melted low and slow, and the marshmallow needs to take on just the perfect golden brown hue. This pursuit of s'more perfection led to the development of this convenient s'mores bar! Make a batch to pack on your next camping trip. The luscious ganache paired with the buttery graham cracker crust and oven-toasted marshmallows will keep you reaching for s'more.

FOR THE GRAHAM CRACKER CRUST

½ cup plus 4 tablespoons (1½ sticks) unsalted butter (168 grams)

1 (14.4-ounce) box graham crackers (408 grams)

¾ teaspoon kosher salt (3 grams)

1 tablespoon confectioners' sugar (10 grams)

½ teaspoon baking powder (2 grams)

FOR THE CHOCOLATE GANACHE

7 ounces chopped dark chocolate (200 grams)

⅔ cup heavy cream (150 grams)

½ teaspoon pure vanilla extract (2 grams)

½ cup (1 stick) plus 1 tablespoon unsalted butter (126 grams)

FOR THE TOPPING

16 large marshmallows (about 105 grams)

1. Preheat the oven to 350°F and line an 8 × 8-inch baking dish with parchment paper, leaving a few inches of overhang on each side so you can easily remove the bars from the pan. Set aside.

2. **Make the crust:** In a medium sauté pan set over medium heat, melt 1½ sticks of the butter. Once the butter is melted, it will begin to foam. Move the pan around a bit to keep it from burning, and allow it to cook until foaming stops, brown bits form on the bottom of the pan, and it smells nutty, 5 to 7 minutes. Remove from heat and let cool slightly.

3. In the bowl of a food processor, add the graham crackers, salt, confectioners' sugar, and baking powder. Pulse until the graham crackers become crushed and resemble sand. Add the brown butter (scraping and including any brown bits from the bottom of the pan) and process until the mixture resembles wet sand and sticks together when you press some between your fingers. Dump the graham cracker mixture into the prepared baking dish and spread into an even layer. Using your hands or the back of a measuring cup, press the crust into a firm, even layer. Bake for 12 to 15 minutes, or until golden brown. Turn off the oven and allow the crust to cool slightly while you make the ganache.

4. **Make the ganache:** In a double boiler, or a large heatproof bowl set over a medium saucepan of simmering water (taking care not to let the bowl touch the water), melt the chocolate until it is completely smooth. Add the heavy cream and vanilla to the bowl and whisk until smooth, shiny, and emulsified. Once emulsified, add the butter to the mixture and whisk until smooth.

5. **Assemble the s'mores:** Pour the ganache over the graham cracker crust, tilting the baking dish slightly to ensure even coverage. Let the ganache set up at room temperature for about 2 hours or until slightly firm to the touch. When the ganache has set, preheat the oven to 400°F.

6. Top the ganache with the marshmallows, leaving some room between each so they can spread under the heat. Place the dish on the top rack of the oven and bake for 5 to 7 minutes, or until the marshmallows are golden brown and toasty.

7. Remove from the oven and let cool to room temperature, then cover and chill in the refrigerator for 6 hours. When ready to serve, run a knife under hot water, wipe off any moisture, and cut the bars into 16 equal-size squares (66 grams each).

Gingerbread Cookies

YIELD: 30 COOKIES

Sorry, Grandma, there's a new gingerbread recipe in town! These cookies have a beautiful soft-baked texture and a refreshing zing from the fresh ginger juice used in the glaze. If you want to give them out as a treat to friends and family during the holidays, I *highly* recommend using a cookie press, which will give them a gorgeous and festive look. Just make sure to label them! If you don't have a press, no worries; you can use the bottom of a sturdy glass or Mason jar to press the dough balls into even rounds.

FOR THE COOKIES

3⅔ cups all-purpose flour (458 grams)

2½ teaspoons ground cinnamon (7 grams)

2½ teaspoons ground ginger (6 grams)

1 teaspoon ground cloves (2 grams)

½ teaspoon ground nutmeg (1 gram)

1 teaspoon kosher salt (6 grams)

¾ teaspoon baking soda (3 grams)

½ cup plus 4 tablespoons (1½ sticks) unsalted butter, at room temperature (168 grams)

½ cup plus 1 tablespoon packed light brown sugar (136g)

⅔ cup pure molasses (240 grams)

2 tablespoons whole milk (28 grams)

FOR THE GINGER ICING

¾ cup confectioners' sugar (98 grams)

2½ tablespoons fresh ginger juice (38 grams) (see Tip)

Pinch of salt (about 1 gram)

1. Preheat the oven to 350°F and line two rimmed baking sheets with parchment paper.

2. Into a medium bowl, sift together the flour, cinnamon, ginger, cloves, nutmeg, salt, and baking soda. Whisk to combine and set aside.

3. In the bowl of a stand mixer fitted with the paddle attachment, add the butter and brown sugar and cream together until pale and fluffy, 3 minutes. Add the molasses and milk and mix on low speed until combined, 1 minute.

4. Scrape down the sides of the bowl and add the flour mixture gradually. Mix on low speed for 1 minute, until just a few streaks of flour remain. Remove the bowl from the stand mixer and fold the dough with a rubber spatula by hand until no streaks of flour remain.

5. Scoop the dough into 30 heaping tablespoon-size dough balls (about 35 grams each) and roll into neat balls. Place the dough balls on the prepared baking sheets, leaving about 4 inches in between each cookie. Using a floured cookie stamp or a floured heavy-bottomed drinking glass, press each dough ball until it is about ¼-inch thick.

6. Bake for 8 to 10 minutes, then transfer the cookies to a wire rack to cool. Repeat with the remaining dough.

7. Make the icing: Into a medium bowl, sift the confectioners' sugar. Add the ginger juice and a pinch of salt and whisk until smooth. Brush the glaze on the cookies while they are still slightly warm. If desired, you can let the first coating of glaze dry, then add an additional coat.

TIP: To make ginger juice, peel and then chop 2 (4-inch) ginger segments into small chunks and add them to a high-speed blender with ½ cup cold water. Blend on high speed for 2 to 3 minutes, or until smooth. Strain through a fine mesh strainer into a storage container and discard the solids.

Horchata Rolls

YIELD: **18 ROLLS**

Los Angeles is obsessed with horchata, for good reason. It is absolutely delicious. A Mexican treasure, horchata can, thankfully, be found in markets across America now. For this recipe you can use store-bought horchata for the glaze, or, if you are feeling spicy, make your own: one cup forbidden rice, one cup water, one tablespoon sugar, and a half teaspoon cinnamon blended and strained. These buns are insanely tender and delicious.

FOR THE DOUGH

¾ cup whole milk, warmed to 110˚F (190 grams)

1 (¼-ounce) packet active dry yeast (7 grams)

1 large egg (50 grams)

1 large egg yolk (18 grams)

½ cup granulated sugar (100 grams)

4 tablespoons unsalted butter, melted (56 grams), plus more for the pans

3⅓ cups bread flour (460 grams)

½ teaspoon kosher salt (3 grams)

FOR THE FILLING

1 cup (2 sticks) unsalted butter (224 grams)

1 cup dark brown sugar (200 grams)

½ cup ground cinnamon (50 grams)

¾ teaspoon kosher salt (4 grams)

½ teaspoon ground ginger (2 grams)

½ teaspoon ground allspice (2 grams)

FOR THE GLAZE

7 ounces cream cheese, softened (200 grams)

2⅓ cups confectioners' sugar (300 grams)

½ cup prepared horchata (110 grams)

1. **Make the dough:** In a small bowl, pour the warm milk over the yeast and gently mix. Let stand for 10 minutes, or until foamy.

2. In a large bowl, whisk the whole egg, egg yolk, and the sugar, mixing for 2 to 3 minutes or until the eggs begin to foam and the sugar starts to dissolve. Whisk in the melted butter until fully incorporated. Add the yeast and milk mixture.

3. Add the bread flour and salt to the liquid mixture and mix with a wooden spoon until a shaggy dough forms. Transfer to a lightly floured surface and knead the dough by hand until smooth, 5 to 8 minutes. The dough should be smooth, shiny, elastic, and not sticky to the touch. If the dough is too sticky, knead a bit more flour into it, 1 tablespoon at a time.

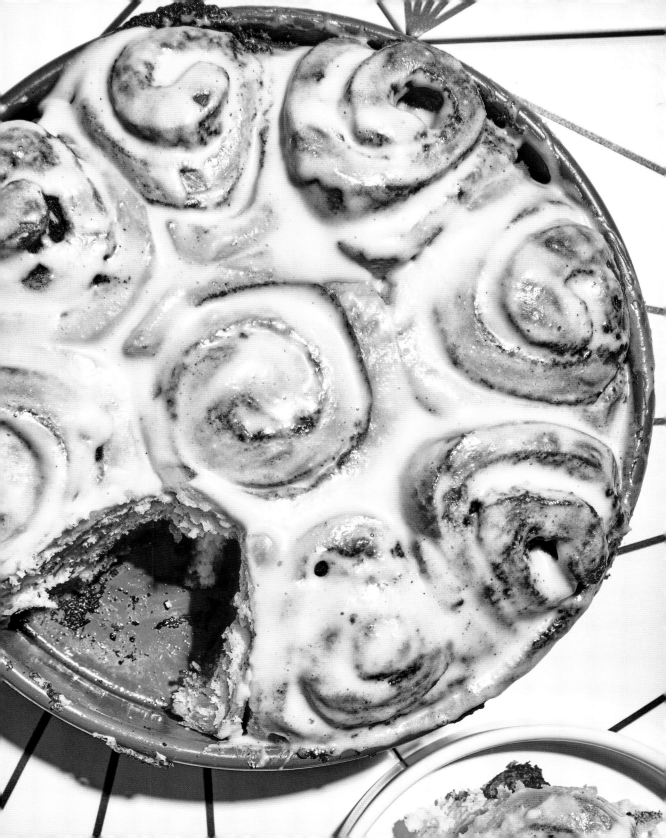

4. Place the dough in a buttered bowl, then cover with a towel or plastic wrap and let rise in a warm spot for 3 hours, or until it has tripled in size.

5. Make the filling: In a medium bowl, whisk the butter, brown sugar, cinnamon, salt, ginger, and allspice. Set aside while the dough proofs.

6. Butter two 9-inch round cake pans and set aside. When the dough has finished rising, punch it down and knead for a few minutes in the bowl to smooth out.

7. On a lightly floured surface, roll out the dough into a 10 × 36-inch rectangle about ¼-inch thick. Dollop the filling across the surface, then spread it into an even layer. Starting with the long end of the dough, roll the dough into a tight spiral, creating a long cylinder. Cut the dough into 2-inch segments, then place 9 rolls, swirl side up, in each prepared pan. Cover and let the dough rise again for about 1 hour, or until the buns puff up and have almost filled the pan.

8. Make the glaze: Add the softened cream cheese to a medium bowl, then work the confectioners' sugar into the cream cheese with a wooden spoon. Add the horchata and whisk until the glaze is smooth.

9. When ready to bake, preheat the oven to 350˚F. Place cake pans on a rimmed sheet pan to catch any drips and bake for 30 minutes, or until golden brown and bubbly. Remove from the oven and let the buns cool slightly before topping with the glaze.

Horchata-Inspired Rice Cereal Treats

YIELD: 16 CEREAL TREATS

Playing off of the incredible rice milk beverage brought to us by the rich culture of Mexico, this riff on a Rice Krispies Treat is the perfect mash-up between the American classic and sweet, creamy, and spicy horchata. With this easy and effortless dessert, I bring to your home a thoughtful and delicious version of what I used to enjoy in college!

½ cup (1 stick) unsalted butter (112 grams), plus more for the pan

½ tablespoon pure vanilla extract (6 grams)

2½ teaspoons ground cinnamon (7 grams)

¾ teaspoon kosher salt (4 grams)

1 (12-ounce) bag marshmallows (350 grams)

4 cups puffed rice cereal (150 grams)

1. Butter an 8-inch square baking pan, then line with two pieces of parchment paper so there is overhang on all four sides, creating a sling you can use to remove the treats.

2. In a double boiler, or in a large heatproof bowl set over a medium saucepan of simmering water (taking care not to let the bowl touch the water), add the butter, vanilla, cinnamon, and salt and cook over the indirect heat until butter is melted, 5 minutes. Add the marshmallows and cook until completely melted, 5 minutes more. Stir the marshmallow and butter mixture together until it is completely combined. Remove from heat.

3. Off the heat, add the puffed rice cereal to the marshmallow mixture and fold in until just combined.

4. Scrape the marshmallow-cereal mixture into the prepared pan, pressing the cereal into an even layer. Cover the pan with the overhanging parchment paper and set in the refrigerator for at least 2 hours before cutting into 16 equal-size squares.

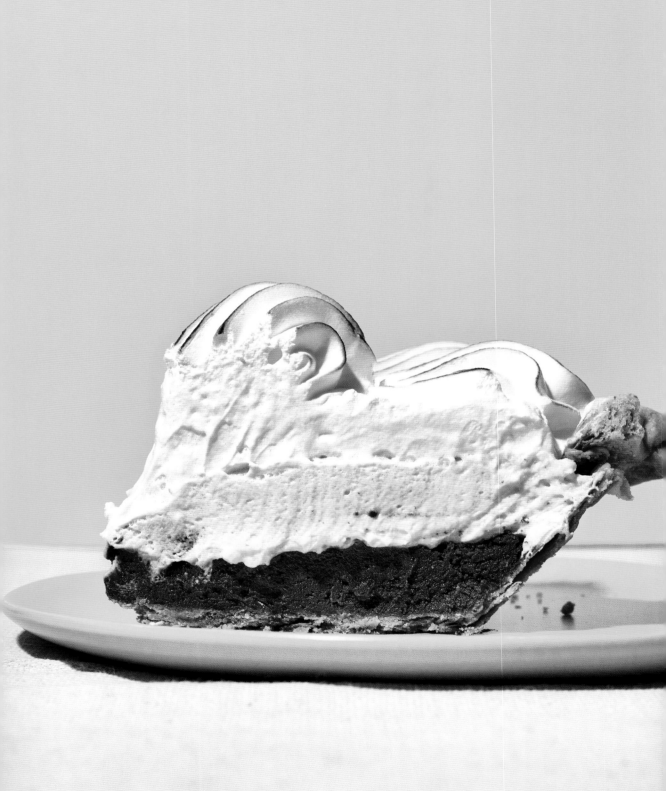

CHAPTER 5

CAKES & PIES

Kabocha Squash Pie

YIELD: **1 (9-INCH) PIE;**
12 SLICES

It's fall, the brisk air is tickling your nose, the wind is brushing against your cheeks, and you pass a bakery or walk into someone's kitchen and catch a waft of sweet pumpkin pie that fills your heart with pure joy and nostalgia. Throw on your comfy socks and an oversized sweatshirt and let's make one of the best fall pies you're ever going to have. Feel free to use a store-bought pie crust if you're in a jam.

FOR THE PIE CRUST

1¼ cups all-purpose flour, plus more for dusting (156 grams)

½ teaspoon kosher salt (2 grams)

3 tablespoons unsalted butter, chilled and cut into small cubes (42 grams)

¼ cup plus 2 tablespoons vegetable shortening, chilled (74 grams)

FOR THE FILLING

2 large eggs (100 grams)

¼ cup packed dark brown sugar (140 grams)

¾ teaspoon ground cinnamon (2 grams)

¼ teaspoon ground allspice

¼ teaspoon ground nutmeg

1 teaspoon pure vanilla extract (4 grams)

⅓ cup heavy cream (150 grams) (see Tip)

1½ cups kabocha puree (705 grams), recipe follows

1. **Make the pie crust:** In the bowl of a food processor, add the flour and salt and pulse to combine. Add the chilled butter and shortening, pulsing the mixture until the flour resembles a coarse meal. Slowly add 2½ tablespoons of ice water until the dough comes together. Do not overmix. Turn the dough out onto a work surface lightly dusted with flour and shape it into a flat, 1-inch-thick disc. Wrap the dough tightly in plastic wrap and refrigerate for at least 30 minutes. If baking right away, preheat the oven to 350°F. The dough can be made ahead and will keep in the refrigerator for up to 2 days.

2. Lightly dust a clean work surface with flour and roll out the dough into a circle, about 12 inches in diameter. Transfer the dough to a 9-inch pie dish, crimping the edges if you wish. Place a sheet of parchment paper on the dough and add pie weights so the crust stays flat while you prebake. Place the pie dish on a sheet pan. Bake for 20 minutes, until the crust is almost fully golden brown. Remove the pie weights and parchment and let the crust cool while you finish the filling.

3. **Make the filling:** In a medium bowl, whisk the eggs and sugar together until pale and fluffy, 3 minutes. Add the cinnamon, allspice, nutmeg, vanilla, and heavy cream to the mixture, and keep whisking until they are fully incorporated. Add the kabocha puree and mix well. Pour the batter into the baked pie crust and bake for 30 to 35 minutes, or until the center is barely set. Let the pie cool completely on a wire rack and serve with whipped cream.

TIP: Add cannabis-infused oil to the heavy cream, whisk until fully incorporated, and continue with recipe.

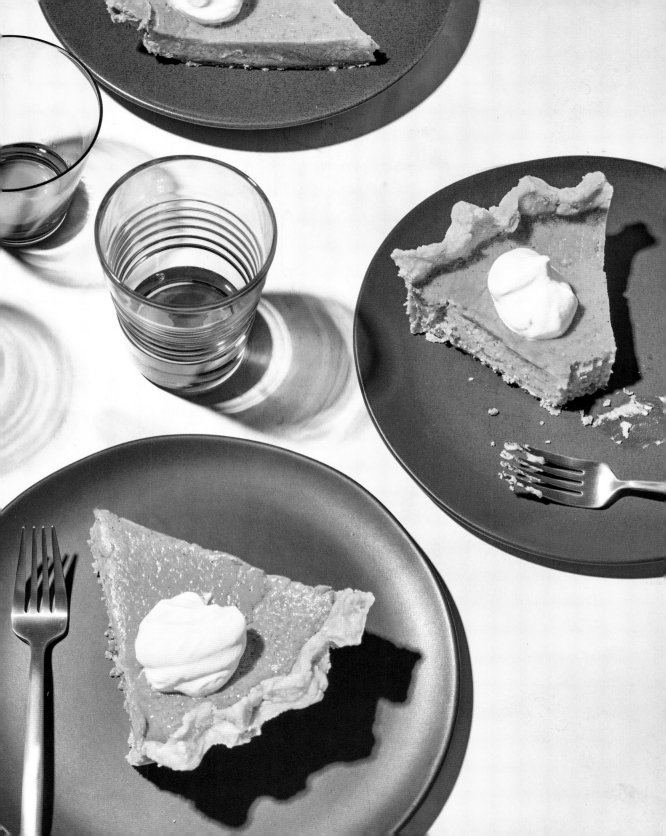

Kabocha Puree

1 small kabocha squash (2½ to 3 pounds)

1 tablespoon avocado oil (14 grams)

¾ cups whole milk (200 grams)

1. Preheat the oven to 350°F and line a baking sheet with parchment paper. Halve the squash vertically and scoop out the seeds of one half; reserve the other half of the squash for another use. Drizzle the oil on the squash and rub all over. Place the squash cut side down on the prepared baking sheet and bake for 45 minutes, or until soft.

2. When the squash is cool enough to handle, scoop out the flesh and set aside. In a medium saucepan, heat the milk over medium heat. Once the milk is warm, add the squash and stir frequently, allowing the milk to soak into the squash until it is completely soft and easily mashes. Use a blender or an immersion blender to puree the mixture. Strain the mixture through a fine mesh strainer.

Confetti Birthday Cake

YIELD: 1 (9-INCH) LAYER CAKE, 12 SLICES

This is sure to hit every part of what you are looking for in a confetti cake. It is moist, light, and has incredible flavor with a fluffy buttercream. Incorporating the whipped egg whites into the cake flour offers more leavening (i.e., lift!) than most cake recipes and yields an incredibly soft birthday cake. I like to use whole milk in this cake because I think the fat content is perfect for the recipe, but if you're looking for a dairy-free alternative, see the Tip. You cannot go wrong with this crowd favorite!

FOR THE CAKE
Nonstick cooking spray, for the pans

1 cup whole milk, at room temperature (244 grams)

6 egg whites, at room temperature (210 grams)

2 teaspoons pure vanilla extract (8 grams)

2¼ cups cake flour, plus more for dusting (202 grams)

2 cups granulated sugar (400 grams)

1½ tablespoons baking powder (16 grams)

¾ teaspoon kosher salt (4 grams)

½ cup plus 4 tablespoons (1½ sticks) unsalted butter, at room temperature (168 grams)

½ cup rainbow sprinkles (80 grams)

FOR THE BUTTERCREAM
1 cup (2 sticks) unsalted butter, at room temperature (224 grams)

2½ cups confectioners' sugar (325 grams)

¼ cup heavy cream (60 grams)

½ teaspoon kosher salt (3 grams)

¼ cup rainbow sprinkles (40 grams), plus more for decorating the cake

1. Preheat the oven to 350°F and move a rack to the middle of the oven. Spray two 9-inch round cake pans with nonstick cooking spray and line the bottoms with parchment paper rounds. Spray the parchment, dust the surfaces with cake flour, and invert the pans and tap to remove excess flour. Set aside.

2. Make the cakes: In a medium bowl, combine the milk, egg whites, and vanilla, then whisk together until well blended.

3. In the bowl of a stand mixer fitted with the paddle attachment, combine the cake flour, sugar, baking powder, and salt over medium speed. Add the butter and beat on low speed until the mixture resembles moist crumbs. Add all but ½ cup of the milk mixture and beat on medium speed until aerated and fluffy, about 1½ minutes. Add remaining ½ cup of the milk mixture and beat 30 seconds more. Scrape down the sides of the bowl with a rubber spatula. Return the mixer to medium speed and beat 20 seconds longer. Fold in the sprinkles with the rubber spatula.

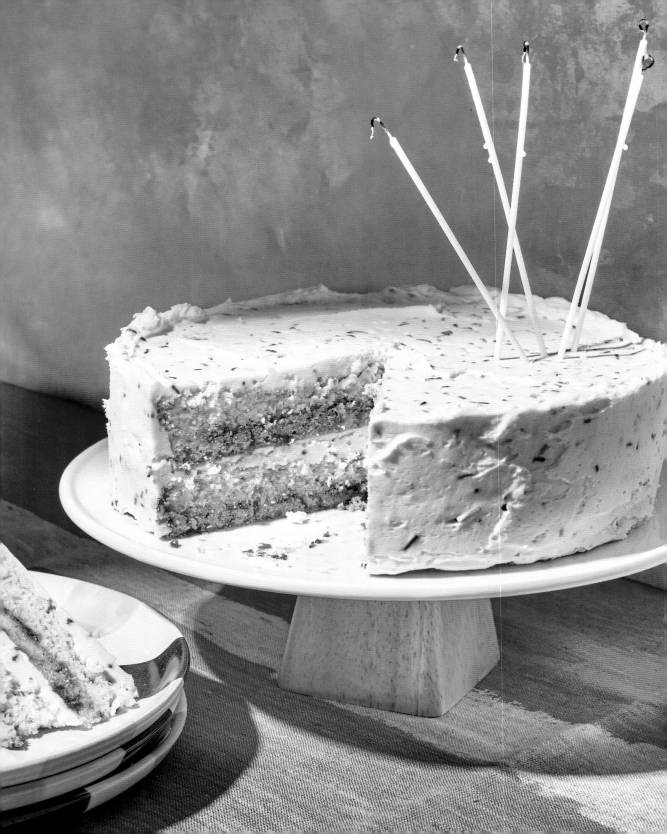

recipe continued

4. Divide the batter evenly between the two prepared pans and smooth the tops with the rubber spatula. Bake for 23 to 25 minutes, or until a toothpick inserted into the center comes out clean. Let cakes rest in pans for 3 to 5 minutes. Loosen each cake from the sides of the pans with a knife and invert onto a wire cooling rack. Let the cakes cool completely, then remove the parchment paper.

5. Make the buttercream: In the bowl of a stand mixer fitted with the paddle attachment, combine the butter, confectioners' sugar, heavy cream, and salt and beat together until very light and fluffy, 4 to 5 minutes. Fold in the sprinkles with a rubber spatula until combined.

6. Assemble the cakes: Once the cakes are completely cooled, transfer one cake round to a plate or cake stand. Top with half of the buttercream. Using an offset spatula, smooth the buttercream into an even layer. Top with the second cake round, and use the remaining buttercream to frost the entire cake. Top with more sprinkles, if desired. Cut into 12 equal-size slices.

TIP: If you are looking for a dairy-free milk alternative, I suggest cashew or macadamia nut milk for the best texture. This recipe uses a reverse creaming technique where you add the butter to the flour mixture, unlike other cake recipes.

Chocolate Cake

YIELD: 1 (9-INCH) CAKE,
12 SLICES

I adore chocolate, which is why you'll see it pretty much everywhere in this book! Baking with chocolate is part of my love language, and this cake is one of my favorites things to bake for the ones I love. The cake is unbelievably light and moist, so bake it for someone you love and tell them it's straight from the heart.

FOR THE CAKE

4 large eggs (200 grams)

3⅓ cups granulated sugar (667 grams)

3 cups cold water (710 grams)

1½ cups avocado oil (327 grams)

1½ teaspoons vanilla bean paste (29 grams)

4½ cups cake flour, plus more for dusting (400 grams)

¾ cup unsweetened cocoa powder (90 grams)

2½ teaspoons baking soda (10 grams)

2 teaspoons kosher salt (12 grams)

Unsalted butter, for the pans

FOR THE CHOCOLATE-ESPRESSO BUTTERCREAM

1 cup (2 sticks) unsalted butter, at room temperature (224 grams)

2½ cups confectioners' sugar (325 grams)

¼ cup heavy cream (60 grams)

½ teaspoon kosher salt (3 grams)

6 ounces dark chocolate, chopped, melted, and cooled but still liquid (113 grams)

1 teaspoon instant espresso powder (5 grams)

1. Preheat the oven to 350°F and line two 9-inch round cake pans with parchment paper, then butter and flour both pans. Set aside.

2. **Make the cakes:** In the bowl of a stand mixer fitted with the whisk attachment, beat the eggs and sugar together until light, fluffy, and pale yellow, 2 to 3 minutes.

3. In a large glass measuring cup or small bowl, add the cold water, avocado oil, and vanilla bean paste.

4. Into a medium bowl, sift together the flour, cocoa powder, baking soda, and salt. With the mixer running on medium speed, alternate adding the dry ingredients and the water-oil mixture to the bowl. Do this in three additions until the ingredients are fully incorporated. Make sure to scrape down the sides of the bowl with a rubber spatula as you go.

5. Scrape the batter into the prepared pans, dividing it evenly between each pan.

6. Bake for 20 to 30 minutes until the cake is set and a cake tester inserted into the center comes out clean. Remove from the oven and let the cakes cool on a wire rack for 15 minutes, then invert onto the rack. Let them cool completely before removing the parchment.

7. **Make the buttercream:** In the bowl of a stand mixer fitted with the paddle attachment, add the butter, confectioners' sugar, heavy cream, and salt and beat together until very light and fluffy, 4 to 5 minutes. Stream in the melted chocolate, add the espresso powder, and mix until combined, 1 to 2 minutes.

8. **Assemble the cakes:** Once the cakes are completely cooled, transfer one cake round to a plate or cake stand, bottom side down. Add a generous dollop of buttercream on top and spread evenly. Top with the second cake round, then frost the entire cake with the remaining buttercream.

Key Lime Pie

YIELD: **1 (9-INCH) PIE,
12 SLICES**

This is my all-time favorite key lime pie. It's silky, light, tangy, and has an incredibly thick graham cracker crust that makes you want to go back for more. Be sure to give yourself enough time to make this before you serve it. It needs to set in the refrigerator for at least six hours, but it is best when it sits overnight. Note: if you can't find key limes, you can swap in the juice of regular limes.

FOR THE CRUST
1 (14.4-ounce) box graham crackers (408 grams)

¾ teaspoon kosher salt (4 grams)

½ cup (1 stick) plus 2 tablespoons unsalted butter, melted (140 grams)

FOR THE FILLING
1 cup granulated sugar (200 grams)

2 large egg yolks (36 grams)

1 cup sour cream (240 grams)

1 cup whole-milk plain Greek yogurt (285 grams)

1 cup canned coconut cream (189 grams)

8 whole key limes, juiced (about 1 cup of juice) (242 grams)

1 (¼-ounce) packet gelatin powder (7 grams)

1. Make the crust: Preheat the oven to 350°F. In the bowl of a food processor, add the graham crackers and salt and pulse until coarse crumbs form. Slowly stream in melted butter while pulsing, until the mixture resembles wet sand.

2. Gently press the mixture into the bottom and sides of a 9-inch pie pan. Bake for 15 minutes, until just golden brown. Set aside to cool.

3. Make the filling: In a large bowl, vigorously whisk the sugar and egg yolks together until light and fluffy. Add the sour cream, Greek yogurt, coconut cream, lime juice, and gelatin. Whisk until they are fully incorporated.

4. Pour the filling into the cooled graham cracker crust and bake until just set but still a little jiggly in the center, 20 to 25 minutes.

5. Let the pie cool, then place it in the refrigerator to set for at least 6 hours or up to overnight before serving. Garnish with thin strips of lime zest if desired.

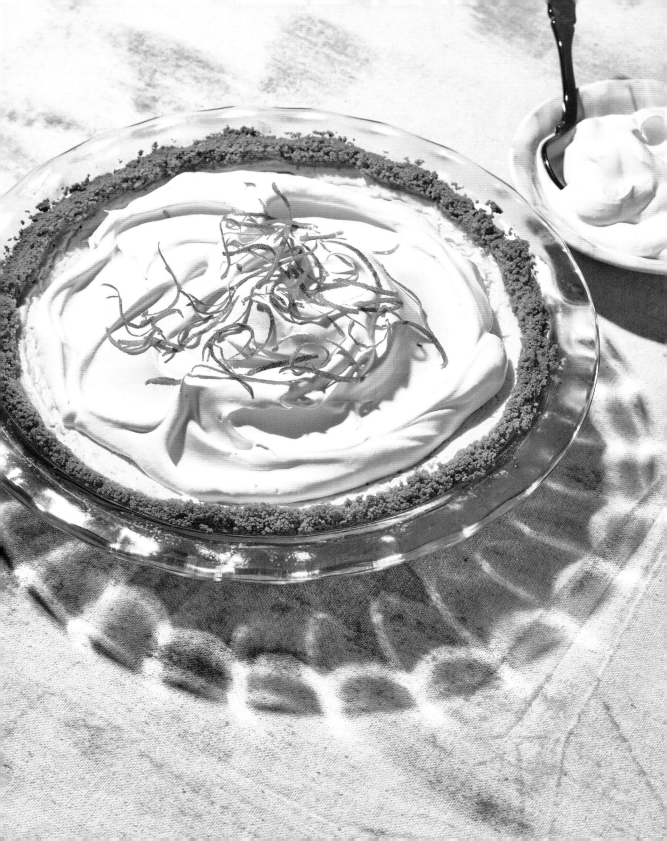

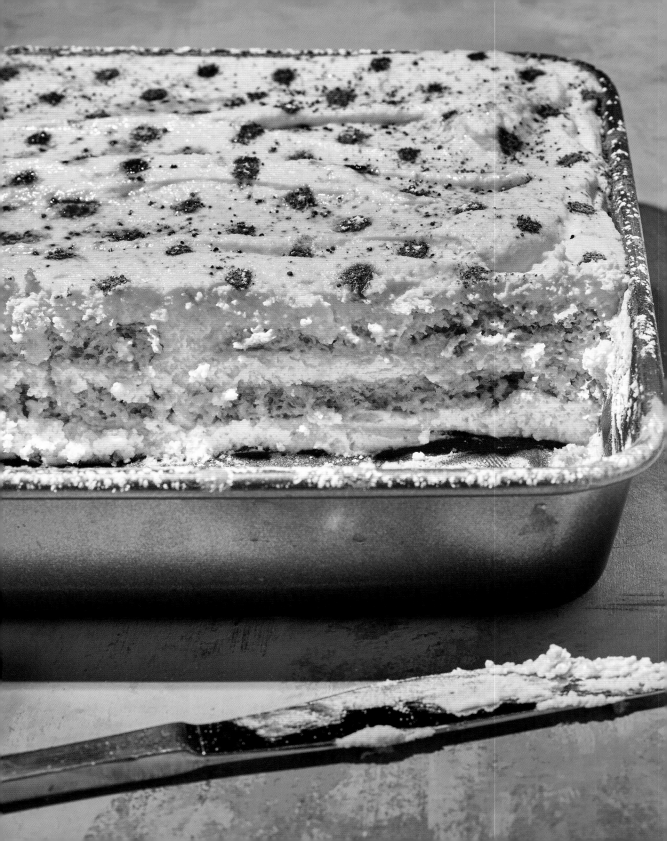

Tiramisu

YIELD: **12 SERVINGS**

Even though I am fully Jordanian, by marriage we have some Italian relatives within my immediate family. And I could not be more grateful for the beautiful blend of cultures and food traditions. My entire life has been a mixture of very loud, vocal, and aggressively loving people, as well as the richest food tapestry you can imagine. This sweet treat is my ode to the Italian side of my family; it's the perfect after-dinner bite, with a lovely hint of espresso and rum.

FOR THE CRÈME ANGLAISE
8 large egg yolks (144 grams)

1 cup granulated sugar (200 grams)

½ cup whole milk (100 grams)

2 teaspoons pure vanilla extract (8 grams)

1 tablespoon brewed espresso (10 grams)

½ teaspoon kosher salt (3 grams)

FOR THE MASCARPONE MOUSSE
3 cups mascarpone cheese, at room temperature (900 grams)

1 cup heavy cream (270 grams)

FOR THE SOAKED LADYFINGERS
40 ladyfinger cookies (340 grams)

⅔ cup brewed espresso (150 grams)

½ cup dark rum (100 grams)

½ cup heavy cream (100 grams)

FOR SERVING
Cocoa powder, as needed

Confectioners' sugar, as needed

1. **Make the crème anglaise:** In a large bowl, whisk together the egg yolks and sugar. Set aside. In a small, heavy-bottomed saucepan, bring the milk to a simmer over medium-low heat. Once simmering, pour the milk over the egg yolk mixture and whisk until thoroughly combined.

2. Return the egg and milk mixture to the saucepan and place over medium heat. Add the vanilla, espresso, and salt and cook, stirring constantly with a heat-safe spatula, until the mixture starts to thicken, 3 minutes. Strain the mixture through a fine mesh strainer into a clean bowl to avoid any clumping, then cover the surface directly with plastic wrap so a film does not form. Place the bowl in the refrigerator to cool.

3. **Make the mascarpone mousse:** Once the crème anglaise has cooled, in a stand mixer fitted with the whisk attachment, add the mascarpone and whip on medium speed until light and fluffy, 2 minutes. Remove the bowl from the stand mixer and fold in the cooled crème anglaise until well combined. Set aside.

4. In the bowl of a stand mixer fitted with the whisk attachment, add the heavy cream and whip on medium speed until soft peaks form. Fold the whipped cream into the mascarpone mixture until well combined.

5. **Soak the ladyfingers:** In a small bowl, combine the espresso, rum, and heavy cream. Dip each side of the ladyfingers into the espresso mixture, then set on a parchment-lined baking sheet.

6. **Assemble the tiramisu:** Spread about 1 inch of the mascarpone mousse into the bottom of a 10 × 10-inch baking dish. Top the cream with a single layer of soaked ladyfingers (you will use about 20 ladyfingers), followed by another inch of cream. Top with one final layer of ladyfingers (about 20 more), then spread remaining cream into an even layer on top. Cover tightly and refrigerate for at least 2 hours.

7. When ready to serve, dust the tiramisu with cocoa powder and confectioners' sugar. Cut the tiramisu into 12 equal-size portions (170 grams).

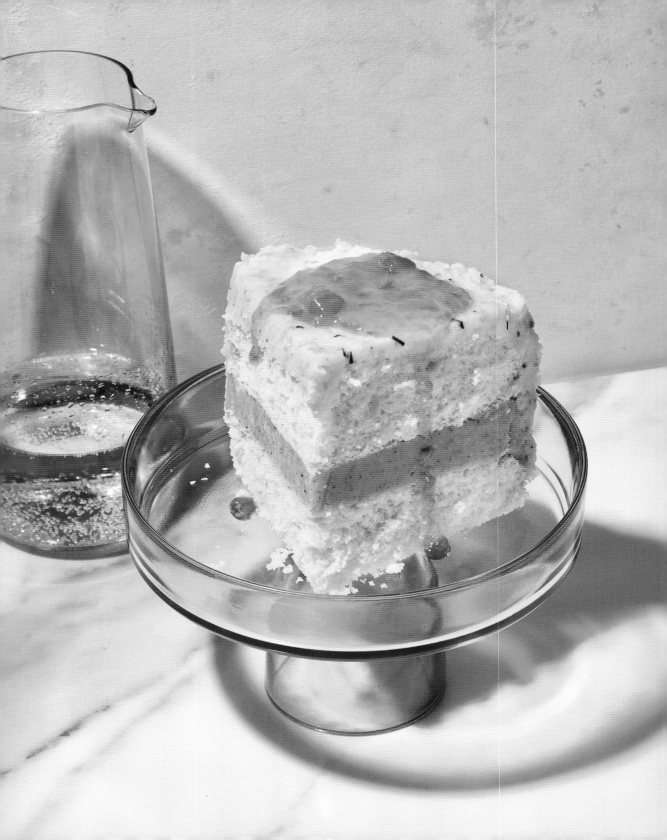

Hemp Oil Cake with Hazelnut Ganache & Apricot Jam

YIELD: **1 (8-INCH) CAKE, 12 SLICES**

This is perfection on a plate. Each ingredient in this recipe works harmoniously with all the others to create one of the most interesting and delicious slices of cake you've ever had. It may not be your average dump-and-mix box cake recipe, but I promise the end result is worth the effort. That said, if you are looking for a few shortcuts, you can make this with a yellow cake mix and substitute hemp oil for the vegetable oil called for on the box recipe. You can also use store-bought apricot jam.

FOR THE CAKE

Nonstick cooking spray, for the pans

¾ cup plus 1 tablespoon granulated sugar, divided (162 grams)

2 large egg yolks (36 grams)

½ tablespoon (3 grams) fresh lemon zest, from ½ medium lemon

2 tablespoons fresh lemon juice (25 grams), from ½ medium lemon

1 teaspoon pure vanilla extract (4 grams)

1 cup minus 1 tablespoon all-purpose flour (113 grams)

¾ cup hemp seed oil (160 grams)

3 large egg whites (105 grams)

½ teaspoon kosher salt (3 grams)

FOR THE HAZELNUT GANACHE

1¼ cups whole hazelnuts (220 grams)

10½ ounces white chocolate, chopped (300 grams)

½ cup (1 stick) plus 6 tablespoons unsalted butter (196 grams)

⅔ cup hemp milk (170 grams)

1 teaspoon pure vanilla extract (4 grams)

FOR THE APRICOT JAM

10 whole apricots, pitted (about 500 grams)

¼ cup honey (85 grams)

¼ teaspoon pure vanilla extract

⅛ teaspoon ground cardamom

⅛ teaspoon white pepper

⅛ teaspoon ground anise

FOR THE ORANGE & TOASTED ROSEMARY BUTTERCREAM

1 tablespoon fresh rosemary leaves (7 grams)

2 cups (4 sticks) unsalted butter, softened (448 grams)

3 tablespoons (15 grams) fresh orange zest, from 3 medium oranges

1½ cups confectioners' sugar (200 grams)

¾ teaspoon kosher salt (4 grams)

½ cup fresh orange juice (50 grams), from 2 medium oranges

½ teaspoon orange extract (2 grams)

recipe continues

1. Preheat the oven to 325°F and line two 8-inch round cake pans with parchment paper and coat with nonstick spray. Set aside.

2. Make the cakes: In a large bowl, whisk ½ cup plus 1 tablespoon of the sugar with the egg yolks until light and fluffy, 2 to 3 minutes. Add the lemon zest, lemon juice, and vanilla and continue to whisk until fully incorporated. Sift the flour into the mixture and fold with a rubber spatula until it is fully incorporated. Switch to a wire whisk and, while whisking constantly, slowly drizzle in the hemp seed oil and mix thoroughly.

3. In the bowl of a stand mixer fitted with the whisk attachment, add the egg whites and beat at medium speed until they form soft peaks, about 3 minutes. Gradually add the remaining sugar and salt and continue whipping the egg whites until they form stiff, shiny peaks, 4 to 5 minutes.

4. Gently fold the egg whites into the flour mixture, taking care not to deflate them. Divide the batter between the two prepared pans and bake for 20 to 25 minutes, or until a toothpick inserted into the center comes out clean. Remove from the oven. (Leave the oven on to roast hazelnuts in the next step.) Cool the cakes on a wire rack for 15 minutes, then invert onto the rack. Once cakes are out of the pans, let them cool completely before removing the parchment and assembling the layer cake.

5. Make the hazelnut ganache: Place the hazelnuts on a rimmed sheet pan and roast in the 325°F oven for 10 minutes, or until nicely toasted. Remove from the oven and let them cool slightly, then place the hazelnuts in a tea towel and rub vigorously to loosen the skins. Discard as much of the skin as possible, then set aside.

6. Place the white chocolate in a heatproof bowl. Then, in a medium saucepan, combine the butter, hemp milk, and vanilla and heat until just simmering. Pour the simmering butter and hemp milk mixture over the chocolate. Cover and let it sit for five minutes. When most of the chocolate has melted, puree with an immersion blender until smooth and shiny. Add the roasted hazelnuts and puree until buttery and smooth. Alternatively, you can transfer the white chocolate mixture and hazelnuts to a high-speed blender and blend until smooth. Set aside to cool to room temperature.

7. Make the apricot jam: In a medium saucepan, combine apricots, honey, vanilla, cardamom, white pepper, and anise. Cover and cook over medium-low heat, stirring occasionally, until the apricots have broken down, 35 to 40 minutes. Puree with an immersion blender or in a high-speed blender, then strain through a fine mesh strainer. Let the jam cool to room temperature.

8. Make the buttercream: Add the rosemary to a dry skillet and toast over medium heat until very fragrant, about 2 minutes. Remove from the heat and finely mince. In the bowl of a stand mixer fitted with the paddle attachment, add the minced rosemary, butter, and orange zest and mix on medium speed until the butter is light and fluffy, 2 to 3 minutes. Add the confectioners' sugar and salt and mix until incorporated. With the mixer running, slowly stream in the orange juice and orange extract and beat for 2 to 3 minutes, or until the buttercream is light and fluffy.

9. Assemble the cakes: Once the cakes are completely cooled, transfer one cake round to a plate or cake stand, bottom side down, then top with the hazelnut ganache. Add the second cake round on top, then frost the whole cake with the prepared buttercream. Cut into 12 equal slices, then drizzle each slice with apricot jam.

Carrot Cake

YIELD: 1 (13 X 9-INCH) CAKE, 8 SLICES

This carrot cake was inspired by my dear friend, who developed a version of it as a special dessert for Javier "Chicharito" Hernández of the LA Galaxy. As the story goes, he enjoyed it so much, he immediately asked for another round! This is a very light version of a traditional carrot cake, just elevated a little bit with spice and a touch of brandy for some zip.

FOR THE CARROT SPONGE CAKE

2 cups superfine almond flour (200 grams)

1 cup confectioners' sugar (125 grams)

2½ teaspoons ground cinnamon (6 grams)

1½ teaspoons ground ginger (4 grams)

½ teaspoon ground allspice (2 grams)

½ teaspoon kosher salt (3 grams)

¼ teaspoon cream of tartar (1 gram)

4 large eggs, at room temperature (200 grams)

2 tablespoons brandy (30 grams)*

1 tablespoon (6 grams) fresh orange zest, from 1 medium orange

2¾ packed cups shredded carrots (about 2 large carrots) (225 grams)

*Add cannabis tincture to brandy and continue with recipe.

FOR THE CREAM CHEESE FROSTING

5 ounces cream cheese, at room temperature (150 grams)

¾ cup confectioners' sugar, sifted (94 grams)

1 teaspoon (5 grams) fresh lemon juice, from ¼ small lemon

¾ teaspoon kosher salt (4 grams)

Carrot sorbet, recipe follows, for serving (optional)

Carrot threads, recipe follows, for garnish (optional)

1. Preheat the oven to 350°F and line a 13 × 9-inch baking dish with parchment paper. Set aside.

2. Make the cakes: Into a large bowl, sift together the almond flour, confectioners' sugar, cinnamon, ginger, allspice, salt, and cream of tartar. Set aside.

3. In a separate large bowl, whisk the eggs, brandy, and orange zest until thoroughly combined, 2 to 3 minutes. Add the carrots to the egg mixture and mix with a wooden spoon to combine.

4. Add the wet ingredients to the dry ingredients and fold until just combined. Scrape the batter into the prepared dish and bake for 15 to 20 minutes, or until a cake tester inserted into the center comes out clean. Remove from the oven and let the cake cool completely on a wire rack. When fully cool, loosen the sides of the cake from the pan with a knife, invert, and place the cake on a serving platter.

5. Make the cream cheese frosting: In a medium bowl, add the cream cheese and whisk for 2 minutes. Add the confectioners' sugar, lemon juice, and salt and continue to whisk until fully incorporated and slightly aerated.

6. Assemble the cake: Cut the sponge cake in half widthwise and spread a generous amount of cream cheese frosting on one side. Put the other half of the sponge on top, then cut the layered cake into 2-inch-thick slices. Put the carrot sorbet on top of each slice, if desired, and then add the carrot threads on top to finish.

recipe continues

Carrot Sorbet

1½ cups granulated sugar (300 grams)

½ cup water (100 grams)

32 ounces carrot juice (1 liter)

1 teaspoon sorbitol (4 grams)

¼ teaspoon kosher salt

1. Add the sugar and water to a small pot and bring to a boil while stirring constantly. Once the syrup reaches a boil, remove from the heat and let cool for 3 minutes.

2. Place the carrot juice in a large bowl and whisk in the sorbet syrup, sorbitol, and salt. Mix thoroughly, then refrigerate for at least 4 hours.

3. In an ice cream maker, churn the chilled sorbet according to the manufacturer's instructions. The sorbet may be soft after it is first churned, so if you prefer you can let it set up in the freezer for a few hours before serving.

Carrot Threads

Avocado oil, as needed for frying

2 medium carrots, peeled, then shredded into long thin threads using a julienne peeler

½ teaspoon kosher salt (2 grams)

1. Line a baking sheet with paper towels. Set aside.

2. Add 2 inches of avocado oil to a wide, deep, heavy-bottomed pot. Using a candy thermometer, heat the oil to 350°F over medium heat. Once the oil reaches the proper temperature, add the carrot threads and fry for 2 minutes. Remove them from the oil with a slotted spoon, sprinkle with the salt, and let drain on the prepared baking sheet.

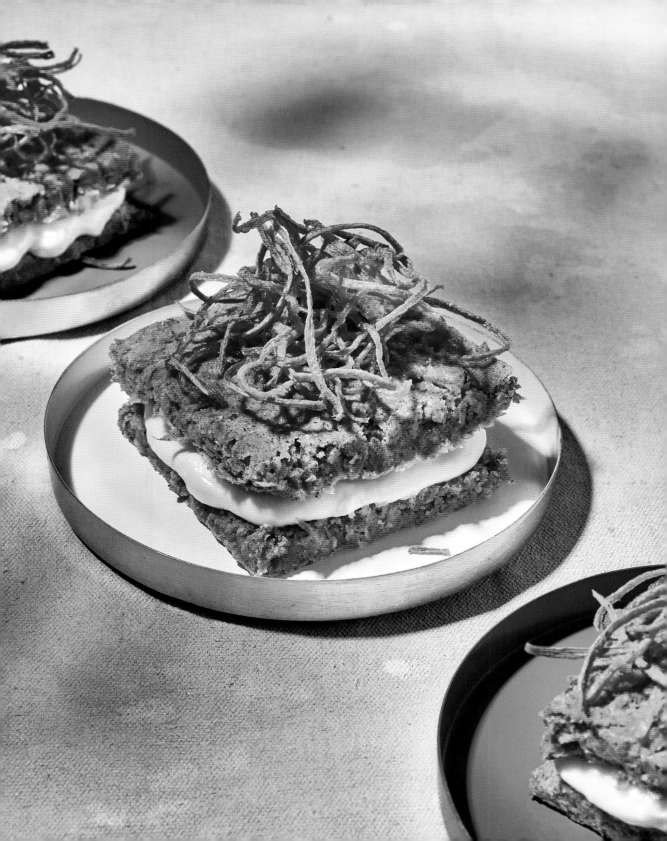

Brown Butter & Thyme Apple Pie

YIELD: 1 (9-INCH) PIE,
12 SLICES

I have always loved apple pie. I mean, who doesn't? However, I've felt like many of the apple pies I've eaten over the years are all more or less the same. The ones that tried to be different were too different and became something else entirely. This apple pie is pretty classic, but a few enhancements put it over the edge into a true autumnal masterpiece. Like any great apple pie, it's best served with vanilla ice cream or chantilly cream (see page 100).

FOR THE PIE CRUST

1¼ cups all-purpose flour, plus more for dusting (156 grams)

½ teaspoon kosher salt (2 grams)

3 tablespoons unsalted butter, chilled and cut into small cubes (42 grams)

⅓ cup vegetable shortening, chilled (74 grams)

FOR THE FILLING

3 tablespoons unsalted butter (42 grams)

1 teaspoon finely chopped fresh thyme leaves (15 grams)

1⅓ cups dark brown sugar (300 grams)

½ teaspoon ground cinnamon (5 grams)

¼ teaspoon ground nutmeg (2 grams)

7 to 8 medium Honey Crisp apples, peeled, cored, and cut into ¼-inch slices (760 grams)

1 teaspoon pure vanilla extract (10 grams)

2 tablespoons all-purpose flour (16 grams)

2 tablespoons (25 grams) fresh lemon juice, from 1 small lemon

FOR THE TOPPING

1 cup raw almond slivers (90 grams)

1 cup old-fashioned oats (90 grams)

2 tablespoons granulated sugar (20 grams)

½ teaspoon kosher salt (3 grams)

½ cup (1 stick) unsalted butter, chilled and cut into cubes (112 grams)

1. **Make the pie crust:** In the bowl of a food processor, add the flour and salt and pulse to combine. Add the cubed cold butter and the shortening in small dollops. Pulse until the mixture resembles a coarse meal with pea-size crumbles. Slowly add 2 tablespoons of ice water until the dough comes together. Do not overmix. Turn the dough out onto a work surface lightly dusted with flour and shape it into a flat, 1-inch-thick disc. Wrap the dough tightly in plastic wrap and refrigerate for at least 30 minutes. If baking right away, preheat the oven to 350°F. The dough can be made ahead and will keep in the refrigerator for up to 2 days.

2. Lightly dust a clean work surface with flour and roll out the dough into a circle, about 12 inches in diameter. Transfer the dough to a 9-inch pie dish, crimping the edges if you wish. Place a sheet of parchment paper on the dough and add pie weights so the crust stays flat while you prebake. Place the pie dish on a sheet pan. Bake until the crust is lightly golden brown, 20 minutes. Remove the pie weights and parchment and let the crust cool while you finish the filling.

3. **Make the filling:** In a large saucepan or Dutch oven, melt the butter over medium-low. Add the thyme and lightly simmer until crisp, about 10 minutes.

4. Add the brown sugar, cinnamon, and nutmeg, stirring to combine. Add the apple slices and vanilla and toss to coat them in the sugar mixture. Let the apples cook down slightly so their juices sweat into the pan while the fruit still retains some crunch, about 10 minutes.

5. Remove the apples with a slotted spoon and spread them on the bottom of the cooled pie crust. While continuing to cook the sugar and brown butter mixture, whisk the flour and lemon juice in a small bowl. Add the flour mixture to the brown butter–sugar mixture and whisk to combine. Simmer until the mixture becomes a thick syrupy consistency, about 5 minutes. Pour over the apples in the pie crust. Set aside while you prepare the topping.

6. **Make the topping:** In a medium bowl, mix almonds, oats, sugar, and salt. Add the butter cubes and use your fingers to press all of the ingredients together while mixing it into the butter. Crumble the topping over the apples in the pie crust and bake until the oat topping is golden brown and the apples are bubbling, 25 minutes. Remove the pie from the oven and let cool at least 30 minutes. Serve with whipped cream or vanilla ice cream.

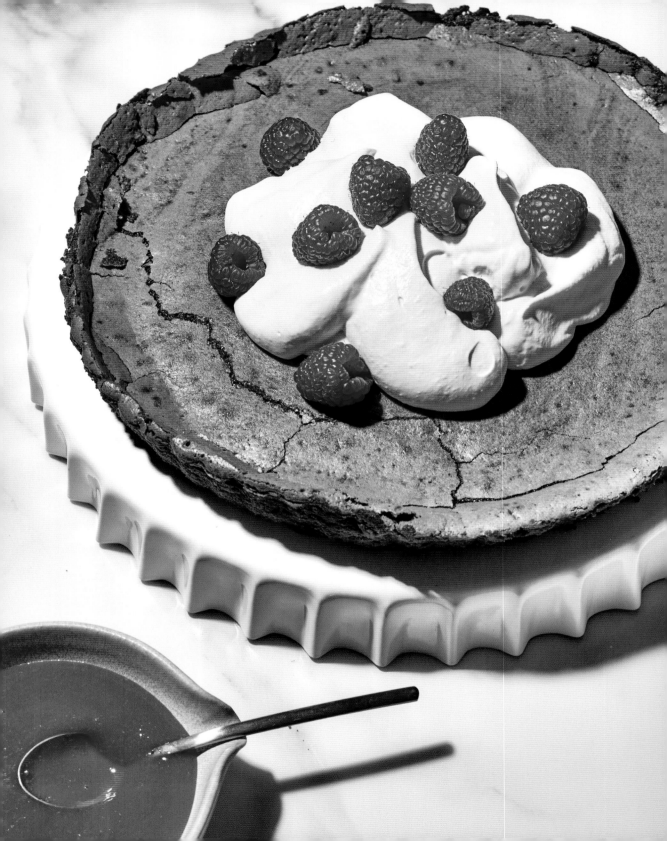

Chocolate-Raspberry Torte

YIELD: 1 (10- OR 11-INCH)
TORTE, 12 SLICES

Some of the best things in the world are in this recipe: chocolate, coconut, and fresh berries. And what makes it even better is the texture. There is a delicate crust atop an incredibly moist flourless cake. The coconut cream and the raspberry coulis lighten the entire dish and balance the decadence with a lovely tangy note of acidity. Break this out for any potluck, and let yourself be known as the dessert whisperer.

FOR THE TORTE
2 cups dark chocolate chips (340 grams)

½ cup (1 stick) plus 3 tablespoons unsalted butter, cut into small cubes (165 grams)

6 large eggs, room temperature (300 grams)

¾ cup granulated sugar (150 grams)

½ teaspoon kosher salt (3 grams)

1 teaspoon pure vanilla extract (4 grams)

FOR THE RASPBERRY COULIS
1 pint fresh raspberries (150 grams)

2 tablespoons (30 grams) fresh lemon juice, from 1 small lemon

¼ cup granulated sugar (50 grams)

Juice and zest of 1 orange (20 grams juice, 8 grams zest)

FOR THE WHIPPED COCONUT CREAM
¾ cup canned coconut cream (150 grams)

¼ cup confectioners' sugar (32 grams)

¼ teaspoon kosher salt

½ teaspoon pure vanilla extract (2 grams)

½ teaspoon (2 grams) fresh lemon juice, from 1 lemon slice

1. Make the cake: Preheat the oven to 350°F and line a 10- or 11-inch tart pan with parchment paper.

2. In a double boiler, or in a medium heat proof bowl set over a small saucepan of simmering water (taking care not to let the bowl touch the water), add the chocolate and stir occasionally with a rubber spatula until completely melted. Add the butter and continue stirring until fully incorporated. Remove from the heat and let it stand for 5 minutes.

3. Meanwhile, in a medium bowl, whisk the eggs, sugar, salt, and vanilla until light and fluffy.

4. Pour the warm chocolate into the egg mixture, mixing with the spatula until everything is incorporated. Add the batter to the prepared pan and bake until the top of the torte is cracking and the center is barely jiggling, 15 to 20 minutes. Let it rest for at least 30 minutes before slicing.

5. Make the coulis: In a medium saucepan over medium-low heat, add the raspberries, lemon juice, sugar, orange juice, and orange zest. Simmer, stirring occasionally, until the berries are completely broken down, about 15 minutes. Let cool slightly, then process the raspberry mixture in a high-speed blender until smooth. Strain through a fine mesh strainer. Allow to cool completely before serving.

6. Make the whipped coconut cream: In the bowl of a stand mixer fitted with the whisk attachment, or in a large bowl with a hand mixer, combine the coconut cream, confectioners' sugar, salt, vanilla, and lemon juice. Whip until light and aerated, about 5 minutes. Top the torte with the coconut cream and a drizzle of the coulis. Slice and serve immediately.

Fluffernutter Pie

YIELD: 1 (9-INCH) PIE;
12 SLICES

For those of you who may feel a bit intimidated by this one, don't! I promise that after you make this, you will have a new favorite pie in your dessert arsenal. This pie is crazy delicious, with so much flavor packed in. If you don't have a kitchen torch, you can use a broiler to caramelize the meringue, but make sure you keep careful watch so it doesn't melt or burn. In the peanut mousse I use a reishi powder; not only is it a great stabilizer, but it has anti-inflammatory healing properties as well.

FOR THE PIE CRUST
1¼ cups all-purpose flour, plus more for dusting (156 grams)

½ teaspoon kosher salt (3 grams)

3 tablespoons unsalted butter, chilled and cut into small cubes (42 grams)

¼ cup plus 2 tablespoons vegetable shortening, chilled and cut into small cubes (74 grams)

FOR THE CHOCOLATE FILLING
1 cup dark chocolate chips (142 grams)

¼ cup heavy cream (50 grams)

4 tablespoons (½ stick) unsalted butter (56 grams)

2 large eggs (100 grams)

⅓ cup plus 1 tablespoon granulated sugar (69 grams)

½ teaspoon kosher salt (3 grams)

½ teaspoon pure vanilla extract (2 grams)

FOR THE PEANUT MOUSSE
1¼ cups heavy cream (250 grams)

⅓ cup confectioners' sugar (65 grams)

1½ tablespoons reishi powder (25 grams) (optional)

¼ cup smooth peanut butter (50 grams)

½ teaspoon pure vanilla extract (2 grams)

FOR THE MARSHMALLOW MERINGUE TOPPING
1 cup granulated sugar (200 grams)

4 large egg whites (140 grams)

½ teaspoon pure vanilla extract (2 grams)

½ teaspoon cream of tartar (2 grams)

1. Preheat the oven to 350°F.

2. Make the pie crust: In the bowl of a food processor, add the flour and salt and pulse to combine. Add the butter and shortening, a little at a time, processing until the mixture resembles a coarse meal. Slowly add a scant tablespoon of water and pulse until the dough comes together. Scrape onto a sheet of plastic wrap and press into an even disc. Wrap the dough and refrigerate for 30 minutes.

3. On a lightly floured surface, roll dough into a 12-inch circle and transfer to a 9-inch pie pan. Trim the excess dough, crimp the edges, and prick the bottom of the crust with the tines of a fork. Set a piece of parchment paper on top of the crust and fill it with dried beans, rice, or pie weights. Blind-bake for 20 to 25 minutes or until the crust is a deep golden brown. Remove the weights and parchment paper and let the crust cool while you prepare the chocolate filling.

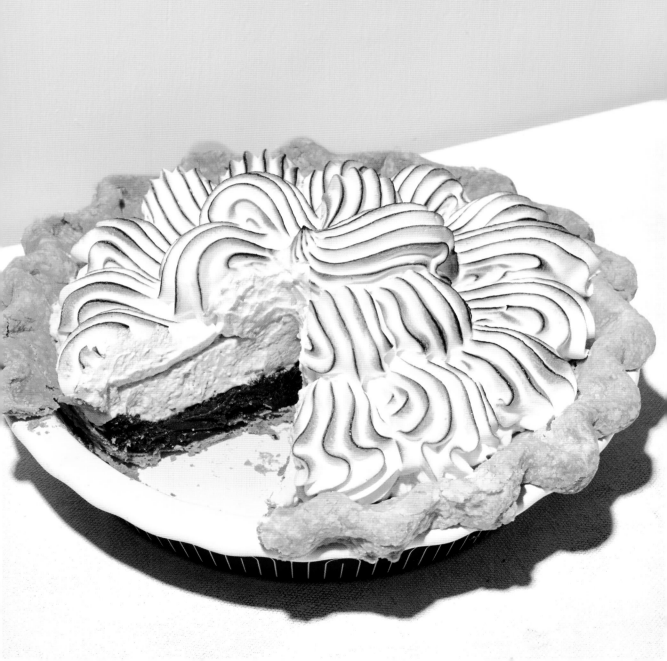

4. Make the chocolate filling:
Keep the oven temperature at 350°F. In a double boiler, or in a large heatproof bowl set over a medium saucepan of simmering water (taking care not to let the bowl touch the water), add the chocolate and stir constantly until melted, 5 minutes. Add the heavy cream and whisk until smooth. Add the butter, stirring until fully incorporated, then remove from the heat and let cool for at least 5 minutes.

5. Meanwhile, in a medium bowl, whisk the eggs, sugar, salt, and vanilla until light and fluffy. Stream the warm chocolate into the egg mixture, mixing with a rubber spatula until everything is incorporated. Add the filling to the cooled pie crust and bake it for 15 to 18 minutes, or until the top is cracked and dry to the touch. Remove from the oven and cool to room temperature, then refrigerate for 1 hour before adding the peanut mousse.

6. Make the peanut mousse:
In a large bowl, whisk the heavy cream, confectioners' sugar, and reishi powder (if using) until it reaches firm stiff peaks and set aside. In a separate large bowl, add the peanut butter and vanilla and stir to loosen up the peanut butter. Add the whipped cream to the peanut butter mixture one large spoonful at a time, folding it gently to combine. Once all the whipped cream has been added, fold the mixture together until no streaks of peanut butter remain and the mixture is light and fluffy. When the pie has chilled, add the peanut mousse on top of the chocolate and smooth it into an even, thick layer. Set in the refrigerator to chill while you make the meringue.

7. Make the meringue: In a small saucepan, add the sugar and ½ cup of water. Bring to a boil, then reduce to a simmer and cook until the sugar has dissolved, 4 minutes. In the clean bowl of a stand mixer fitted with the whisk attachment, add the egg whites and whisk on low speed for 2 minutes. Gradually increase the speed until the egg whites start to foam. Add the vanilla and cream of tartar and whip until soft peaks form, 4 to 5 minutes. Increase the mixer speed to high and carefully add the warm sugar syrup in a thin, even stream. Once all the sugar syrup has been added, continue to whisk until the meringue begins to cool and is bright white and shiny. Transfer the meringue to a pastry bag or sturdy zip-top bag and pipe on top of the peanut mousse. Using a culinary torch (if desired) torch the peaks of the marshmallow meringue and serve.

Parsnip Funnel Cake

YIELD: **4 LARGE FUNNEL CAKES**

I love to hide vegetables in pretty much everything. They are deliciously versatile, and I want everyone to taste their glory and be surprised by how much they enjoy them! Parsnip has some very sweet notes and is a great base for cakes. This cake will work with any squash or root vegetable, so get creative!

2 medium parsnips, peeled and sliced into coins (160 grams)

1 cup water (250 grams)

2 large eggs (100 grams)

¼ cup granulated sugar (50 grams)

⅔ cup whole milk (160 grams)

1 teaspoon pure vanilla extract (4 grams)

2 cups all-purpose flour (250 grams)

¾ teaspoon baking powder (3 grams)

½ teaspoon ground cinnamon (2 grams)

⅛ teaspoon ground nutmeg

¾ teaspoon kosher salt (4 grams)

Avocado oil, as needed for frying (about 24 fluid ounces)

Confectioners' sugar, for dusting

1. In a small saucepan over medium-high heat, add the parsnips and water and bring to a boil. Reduce the heat to a simmer and cook for about 20 minutes, or until the parsnips are very soft and can be mashed with a fork.

2. Remove the parsnips from the heat and place in a high-speed blender. Blend on high speed for 1 to 2 minutes, adding water 1 tablespoon at a time as needed, until you get a silky smooth puree. You should have about ¾ cup of puree. Set aside to cool completely.

3. Once the puree is cool, add the eggs and sugar to a large bowl and whisk for 2 minutes, or until light and fluffy. Add the parsnip puree, milk, and vanilla and mix thoroughly until fully incorporated. Set aside.

4. In a separate medium bowl, sift together the flour, baking powder, cinnamon, nutmeg, and salt, then whisk until combined. Add the dry ingredients to the wet ingredients in three additions, folding just until no streaks of flour remain. Scrape the batter into a pastry bag or sturdy zip-top bag and refrigerate for 30 minutes.

5. While the batter chills, add the oil to a medium heavy-bottomed, deep-sided pot. The oil should come 3 to 4 inches up the side of the pot. Fix a candy thermometer to the side of the pot and bring the oil to 350°F. Place a wire rack on a paper towel–lined sheet pan and set aside.

6. Once the oil reaches the proper temperature, snip a hole in the corner of the bag and pipe the batter into the hot oil in large concentric circles. Use about ¼ of the batter for each funnel cake. Cook for 3 minutes, then carefully flip and cook on the other side for 2 to 3 minutes more. Remove the funnel cake from the hot oil and let it drain on the rack set over the prepared sheet pan.

7. Repeat with the remaining batter. You should make about 4 large funnel cakes in total. Drain and let cool slightly, then dust with confectioners' sugar and serve warm.

TIP: You can top this recipe with Strawberry Glaze, Chocolate Glaze, or Maple Glaze (p. 120)!

Strawberry Shortcake

YIELD: **10 SHORTCAKES**

I love a simple recipe as much as I love a challenge. This is one of the simplest dishes I know—and also one of my favorite crowd-pleasers. Can't beat that. The most important factor in making this cake is not to overmix the biscuit dough. For the lightest, fluffiest biscuits, mix the dough until it just comes together and then stop. There's really not much to this cake, so be sure to use the very best berries you can find. If you see me at the Santa Monica farmers market picking up berries, don't be afraid to say hello.

FOR THE BISCUITS

2¾ cups all-purpose flour (344 grams)

1 tablespoon baking powder (12 grams)

¾ teaspoon kosher salt (4 grams)

¾ cup plus 2 tablespoons unsalted butter, chilled and cut into small cubes, divided (196 grams)

¾ cup cold buttermilk (183 grams)

2 tablespoons honey (43 grams)

FOR THE MACERATED STRAWBERRIES

1 pound strawberries, hulled and quartered (about 3 cups) (454 grams)

⅓ cup granulated sugar (66 grams)

2 tablespoons (30 grams) fresh lemon juice, from 1 small lemon

2 tablespoons fresh orange zest (12 grams), from 2 medium oranges

FOR THE WHIPPED CREAM

1 cup heavy cream (235 grams)

¼ cup confectioners' sugar (33 grams)

1 teaspoon pure vanilla extract (4 grams)

½ teaspoon ground nutmeg, plus more for garnish (3 grams)

2 tablespoons (23 grams) fresh orange juice, from ½ medium orange

1. **Make the biscuits:** In the bowl of a food processor, add the flour, baking powder, and salt and pulse to combine. Add ¾ cup of the butter and pulse until it resembles coarse sand. Add the buttermilk and honey and pulse until the dough just comes together, no more than 30 seconds. Do not overmix or you will end up with tough biscuits. Turn the dough out onto plastic wrap and shape it into a flat disc. Refrigerate the dough for at least 45 minutes.

2. Preheat the oven to 375°F and line a rimmed baking sheet with parchment paper. Take the dough out of the refrigerator and roll it into a 1-inch-thick circle. Using a 3-inch round cookie cutter or the mouth of a glass, cut out biscuits and arrange them on the prepared baking sheet about 1 inch apart. Reroll any scraps and cut more circles until you have 10 biscuits. Melt the remaining 2 tablespoons of butter. Brush the tops of the biscuits with the melted butter and bake until golden brown, 15 to 17 minutes. Let cool and set aside for assembly.

3. **Make the macerated strawberries:** In a large bowl, toss the strawberries with the sugar, lemon juice, and orange zest. Set aside for at least 20 minutes, or until the juices pool.

4. **Make the whipped cream:** In the bowl of a stand mixer fitted with the whisk attachment, or with a hand mixer in a medium bowl, whip the heavy cream and confectioners' sugar on medium speed until soft peaks form. Add the vanilla and nutmeg and then very slowly add the orange juice. Cover and refrigerate until ready to use.

5. To assemble, cut each biscuit in half. On the bottom half, mound some of the macerated strawberries with their juices, then some of the whipped cream, then the other half of the biscuit. Top again with strawberries and cream. Add some nutmeg on top as a garnish.

TIP: Any extra dough can be wrapped and saved in the freezer for up to 9 months.

GOAT Cheesecake

YIELD: **1 (9-INCH) CAKE,
12 SLICES**

This is one of my all-time favorite cheesecake recipes because it offers the perfect balance between sweet and tart. As with any cheesecake, be gentle here; make sure there is still a little jiggle when it comes out of the oven and let it set fully, even overnight. Remember, the thicker the crust, the better.

FOR THE CRUST

18 chocolate crème–filled sandwich cookies (I use Newman's Own) (245 grams)

2 tablespoons granulated sugar (25 grams)

6 tablespoons unsalted butter, (84 grams)

FOR THE FILLING

8 ounces cream cheese, at room temperature (225 grams)

1 (8-ounce) log goat cheese, at room temperature (230 grams)

⅓ cup crème fraîche, at room temperature (80 grams)

1 cup granulated sugar (200 grams)

¼ teaspoon kosher salt (2 grams)

1 teaspoon pure vanilla extract (4 grams)*

4 large eggs, at room temperature (200 grams)

* Add cannabis tincture to vanilla and continue with recipe.

1. Preheat the oven to 325°F. Place one rack in the middle of the oven and another rack in the lower third of the oven. Line a 9-inch springform pan with aluminum foil. Set aside.

2. Make the crust: In the bowl of a food processor, add the cookies and sugar and pulse to combine. Add the melted butter and process until the mixture resembles wet sand. Press the cookie mixture into the bottom of the prepared pan until it is about ½-inch thick.

3. Make the filling: In the bowl of a stand mixer fitted with the whisk attachment, whip the cream cheese, goat cheese, and crème fraîche on medium speed until aerated and fluffy, about 4 minutes. Add the sugar, salt, and vanilla and continue to mix. Add the eggs, one at a time, until fully combined. Pour the cheesecake batter into the pan with the crust.

4. Fill a 13 × 9-inch pan one-third of the way with boiling water. Set the cheesecake on the middle rack of the oven and place the pan with water on the lower rack. Bake until the center barely jiggles, 35 to 40 minutes.

5. Turn the oven off and crack the door open. Allow the cheesecake to rest in the oven for 20 minutes. This will prevent cracks from forming on top of the cheesecake. Remove the cake from the oven and let it cool for another 45 minutes before refrigerating to cool completely, about 5 hours. Carefully release the cheesecake from the springform pan and slice.

Cherry Custard Loaf

The beauty of this cake is that it can be riffed on infinitely. Want nuts? Add them. Want more chocolate? Why not! Dried fruit? Toss some in. This gluten-free cake is the perfect base for your favorite flavors and add-ins.

4 cups cherries (fresh or frozen), pitted and divided (560 grams)

1 cup whole-milk yogurt (270 grams)

1 cup almond milk (250 grams)

½ teaspoon (2 grams) fresh lemon juice, from 1 lemon slice

½ cup pure maple syrup (180 grams)

1 cup coconut cream (250 grams)

2¼ cups cassava flour (300 grams)

3 tablespoons baking powder (37 grams)

½ teaspoon kosher salt (3 grams)

2 cups dark chocolate chips (230 grams)

1. In a high-speed blender, place 3 cups of cherries and blend on high until you have a smooth puree. Strain through a fine mesh strainer and set aside.

2. Preheat the oven to 350°F and line a 13 × 9-inch baking dish with parchment paper. In a large bowl, whisk together 1½ cups of the cherry puree with the yogurt, almond milk, lemon juice, maple syrup, and coconut cream. Into a separate medium bowl, sift together the cassava flour, baking powder, and salt. Add a third of the wet mixture to the dry ingredients and mix just to combine. Repeat with the remaining wet ingredients, a third at a time. Fold in the dark chocolate chips.

3. Pour the mixture into the prepared baking dish. Halve the remaining 1 cup of cherries and scatter them across the top of the batter. Bake until a toothpick inserted into the center comes out clean, 25 to 30 minutes. Let it cool slightly, then slice.

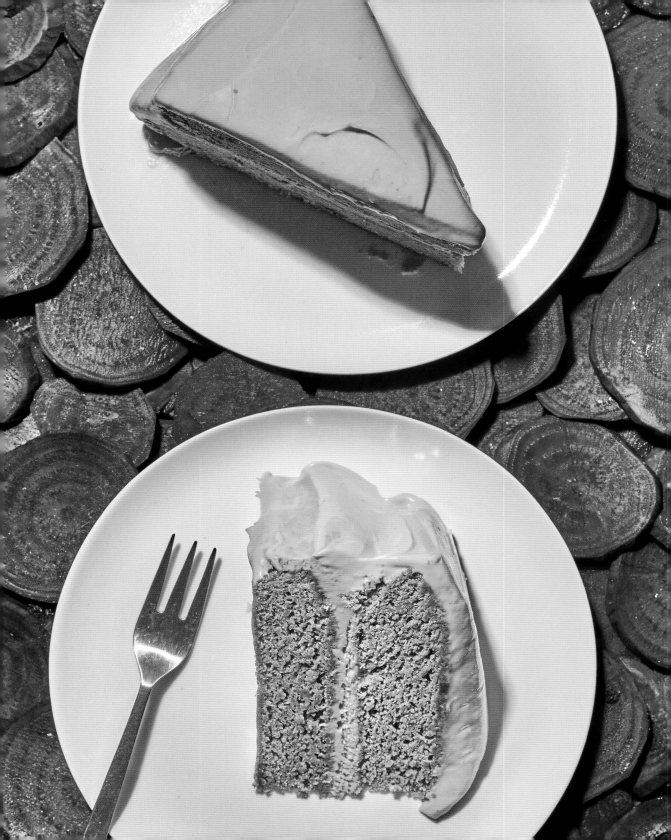

Beet Root Cake

Everyone has a red velvet cake, right? Many traditional recipes use food coloring, which is not ideal. My version, however, is made with beets, which make this cake especially delicious all while using natural flavors and colors. The red beet juice not only gives this cake a gorgeous color, it also lends it an earthiness and moisture.

FOR THE CAKE

Nonstick cooking spray or butter, for the pans

2⅔ cups all-purpose flour (333 grams)

2 tablespoons cocoa powder (14 grams)

1 teaspoon baking powder (4 grams)

1 teaspoon kosher salt (6 grams)

1 cup avocado oil (200 grams)

2½ cups granulated sugar (450 grams)

2 large eggs, at room temperature (100 grams)

½ cup beet juice (118 grams)

1 tablespoon pure vanilla extract (12 grams)

½ cup hot coffee (109 grams)

FOR THE CREAM CHEESE FROSTING

12 ounces cream cheese, softened (352 grams)

½ cup plus 1 tablespoon mascarpone cheese, softened (100 grams)

2 cups confectioners' sugar (260 grams)

2 teaspoons pure vanilla extract (8 grams)

¼ cup beet juice (60 grams)

1 tablespoon (15 grams) fresh lemon juice, from ½ small lemon

1. Preheat the oven to 350°F. Line two 9-inch round cake pans with parchment paper, then grease with nonstick cooking spray or butter. Set aside.

2. Make the cakes: Into a medium bowl, sift together the flour, cocoa powder, baking powder, and salt, then whisk to combine. Set aside.

3. In the bowl of a stand mixer fitted with the paddle attachment, add the oil and granulated sugar and beat on medium speed until well combined, 1 to 2 minutes. Beat in the eggs one at a time. Then, with the machine on low speed, very slowly add the beet juice and vanilla. Add the flour mixture in two batches to the egg mixture, alternating with the hot coffee. Scrape down the sides of the bowl and mix just until no streaks of flour remain.

4. Divide the batter evenly between the prepared pans and bake for 30 minutes, or until a toothpick inserted into the center comes out clean. Let the layers cool in their pans on a wire rack for 20 minutes, then invert onto the rack. Allow the layers to cool completely while you make the cream cheese frosting.

5. Make the frosting: In the bowl of a stand mixer fitted with the paddle attachment, add the cream cheese, mascarpone cheese, confectioners' sugar, vanilla, beet juice, and lemon juice and beat until light and creamy, 3 to 4 minutes.

6. Assemble the cakes: Once the cakes are completely cooled, remove the parchment paper liners and transfer one cake layer to a plate or cake stand, bottom side down. Top with a generous dollop of frosting and spread evenly, then place the remaining cake layer on top. Frost the entire cake with the remaining frosting.

Pecan Pie

YIELD: **1 (9-INCH) PIE, 8 SLICES**

If you haven't noticed, I am a big crust guy. This is a deep dish–style pecan pie that gets a little kick from bourbon and Grand Marnier. It is deliciously ooey and gooey. I like to top mine with a little fleur de sel and whipped cream. I hope you love it!

FOR THE CRUST

1¼ cups all-purpose flour (156 grams), plus more for dusting

½ teaspoon kosher salt (3 grams)

3 tablespoons unsalted butter, chilled and cut into cubes (42 grams)

¼ cup plus 2 tablespoons vegetable shortening, chilled (74 grams)

FOR THE FILLING

6 large eggs (300 grams)

2 large egg yolks (36 grams)

½ cup (1 stick) unsalted butter, melted (112 grams)

1 cup inverted sugar or light corn syrup (350 grams)

2 cups brown sugar (440 grams)

1 tablespoon vanilla bean paste (19 grams)

1 tablespoon kosher salt (18 grams)

1 tablespoon bourbon (15 grams)

1 tablespoon Grand Marnier (15 grams)

2 cups shelled pecans (245 grams)

FOR THE WHIPPED CREAM

1 cup heavy cream (235 grams)

1 teaspoon freshly grated nutmeg (6 grams)

½ cup plus 1 tablespoon confectioners' sugar (73 grams)

1 teaspoon pure vanilla extract (4 grams)

½ teaspoon bourbon (3 grams)

1. Make the pie crust: In the bowl of a food processor, add the flour and salt. Add the butter and shortening and pulse the mixture until the flour resembles a coarse meal. Slowly add 2½ tablespoons of ice water until the dough comes together. Turn the dough out onto a work surface and shape it into a flat, 1-inch-thick disc. Wrap the dough in plastic and refrigerate it for at least 30 minutes.

2. When ready to bake, preheat oven to 350°F and line a 9-inch springform pan with parchment paper. Lightly dust a clean work surface with flour and roll out the dough into a 12-inch circle. Transfer the dough to the prepared pan. Allow some of the crust to hang over the edge, but not more than half an inch down the side of the pan.

3. Make the filling: In a medium bowl, whisk the eggs, egg yolks, butter, inverted sugar, brown sugar, vanilla bean paste, salt, bourbon, and Grand Marnier. Once fully incorporated, add the pecans and mix thoroughly. Pour the filling into the pie crust.

4. Bake the pie until the crust is golden and the middle of the pie barely jiggles, 75 to 90 minutes. Let the pie rest for at least 1 hour before slicing.

5. Make the whipped cream: In a medium bowl, add the heavy cream, nutmeg, and confectioners' sugar and whisk until firm peaks form. Add the vanilla and bourbon and whisk again. Serve the whipped cream over the cooled pecan pie.

Pear-Frangipane Tart

YIELD: **1 (10-INCH) TART,
8 SLICES**

This is definitely one of my all-time favorite desserts because it is not too sweet. It relies on the pears for sweetness and flavor. I use Red Bartlett pears, and I don't think you can go wrong with those. But you can swap them out for another pear variety or quince. Just make sure to adjust the cooking time if they are bigger than your average pear. They should be mostly soft to the core with a little resistance, as they will continue cooking in the oven. You'll use about half of your dough, and you can wrap and store the rest in the freezer for round two.

FOR THE TART DOUGH

3¾ cups all-purpose flour, plus more for dusting (469 grams)

1½ cups (3 sticks) unsalted butter, chilled and cut into cubes (336 grams)

4½ tablespoons coconut nectar, also referred to as coconut sap (84 grams)

3 teaspoons kosher salt (18 grams)

3 large eggs (150 grams)

FOR THE FILLING

3 Bartlett pears, peeled (215 grams)

1½ liters pomegranate juice (1.4 kilograms)

2 cinnamon sticks

2 sprigs fresh mint

Zest and juice of 1 orange (15 grams of juice, 2 grams of zest)

3 black peppercorns

1 whole star anise

FOR THE FRANGIPANE

½ cup (1 stick) unsalted butter (112 grams)

½ cup plus 1 tablespoon maple syrup (196 grams)

2 large eggs, at room temperature (100 grams)

1 teaspoon pure vanilla extract (4 grams)

1 teaspoon almond extract (4 grams)

3 tablespoons peach preserves (46 grams)

1 tablespoon Grand Marnier (16 grams) (optional)

1 cup almond flour (85 grams)

¼ teaspoon kosher salt (3 grams)

2 tablespoons all-purpose flour (19 grams)

2 tablespoons sliced almonds, toasted (25 grams)

1. **Make the tart dough:** Into a large bowl, sift the flour and add butter. Gently work the butter into the flour with a pastry cutter or your hands until it is crumbly. Set aside.

2. In a small bowl, combine the coconut nectar, salt, and eggs and mix well. Add the egg mixture to the flour mixture and knead it into a dough. Divide the dough into two large, flat discs and wrap them in plastic wrap (you will only use one disc for this recipe, so you can freeze the other disc for future use, up to 9 months). Refrigerate the dough for at least 30 minutes or up to 2 days.

recipe continues

3. When ready to bake, preheat the oven to 375°F. Roll one tart dough disc out on a lightly floured surface to ¼-inch thick. Place the dough over a 10-inch tart pan and gently push the dough into the shell and up the sides of the pan. Trim any excess dough. Use the tines of a fork to make a few indentations on the bottom of the dough. Place the tart pan on a sheet pan and place a sheet of parchment over the dough. Weigh down the parchment with pie weights. Blind-bake until slightly golden, 12 to 15 minutes. Remove the parchment with pie weights and allow the crust to cool completely while you assemble the rest of the dish.

4. **Make the filling:** In a large saucepan over low heat, combine the pears, pomegranate juice, cinnamon sticks, mint, orange zest, orange juice, black peppercorns, and star anise. Bring the liquid to a simmer and let it cook until the pears are dark red and tender all the way through, 90 minutes. Turn off the heat and let the pears cool completely in the liquid. Once cooled, use tongs to remove the pears. Place the saucepan with the remaining liquid over medium-high heat and cook until reduced by 75 to 80 percent, or until it resembles a syrup consistency. Let cool.

5. **Make the frangipane:** In the bowl of a stand mixer fitted with the paddle attachment, cream the butter and maple syrup on medium speed until combined. Add the eggs, one at a time, and mix until fully incorporated. Add the vanilla, almond extract, peach preserves, and Grand Marnier and mix until incorporated, scraping down the bowl as needed. Add the almond flour salt, and all-purpose flour to the mixture. Mix until combined.

6. **Assemble the tart:** Using an offset or rubber spatula, spread the frangipane evenly on the bottom of the cooled tart shell.

7. Cut the cooled poached pears in half vertically and remove the cores. With the pear halves cut side down, thinly slice them width-wise. Place the pear slices on top of the frangipane. Bake until the tart shell and frangipane are golden brown, 45 minutes.

8. Place the tart on a wire rack to cool completely. Brush the pears with the pomegranate syrup and top with the sliced almonds. Slice and serve immediately.

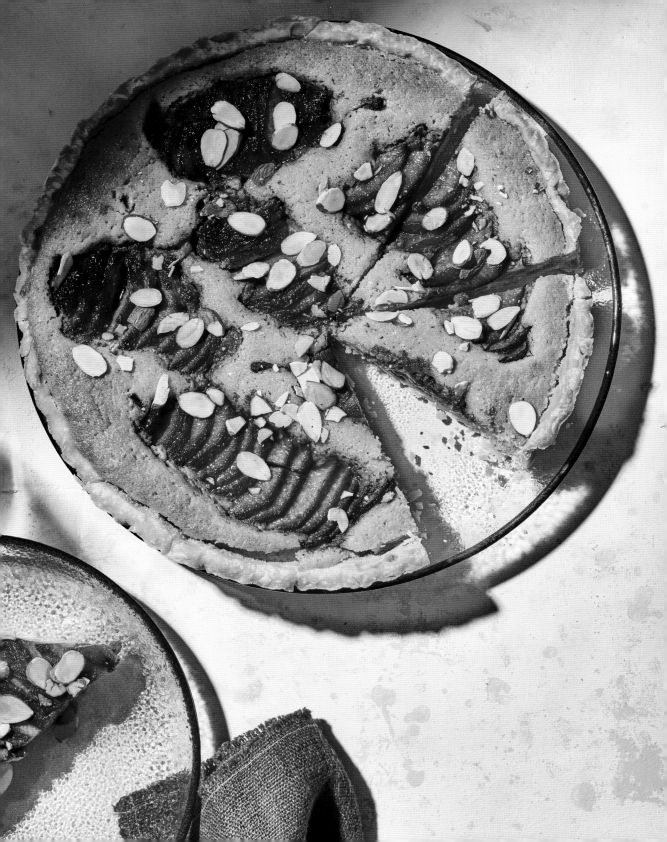

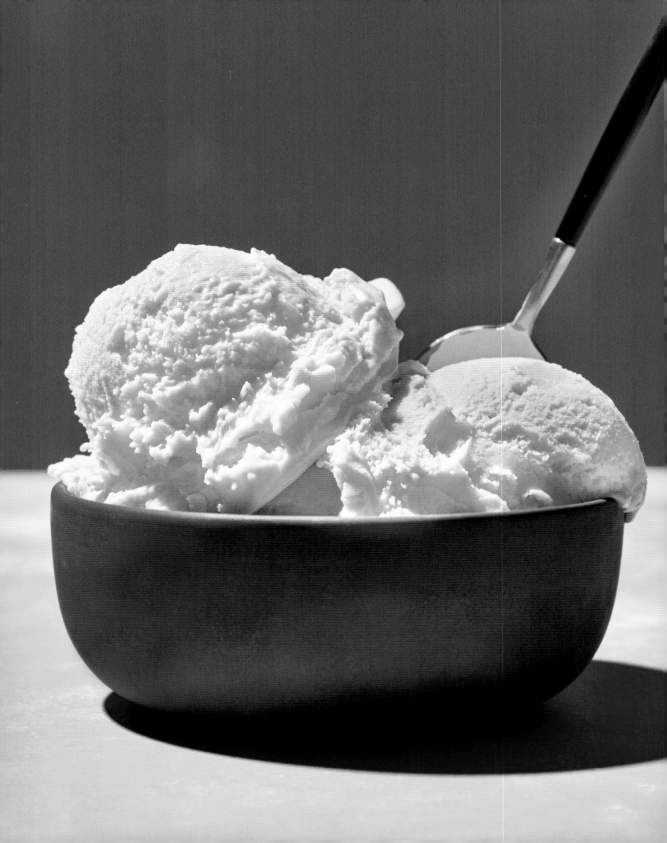

CHAPTER 6
MISCELLANEOUS SWEET TREATS

Chocolate Custard

This ethereal chocolate custard is sweetened with pure maple syrup and is the ultimate make-ahead dessert. Whip up a batch to stash in the refrigerator for the week ahead—my kind of meal prep!

1¾ cup dark chocolate chips (283 grams)

1¼ cups coconut cream (310 grams)

1 large egg yolk (18 grams)

2½ tablespoons pure maple syrup (54 grams)

1 tablespoon chocolate collagen peptide powder (9 grams)

1 teaspoon pure vanilla extract (4 grams)

1 egg white (35 grams)

1 tablespoon honey (20 grams)

1. In a double boiler, or in a medium heatproof bowl set over a small saucepan of simmering water (taking care not to let the bowl touch the water), add the chocolate chips and melt completely. Remove from the heat and set aside to cool.

2. In a medium saucepan over low heat, add the coconut cream, egg yolk, maple syrup, chocolate collagen powder, and vanilla and whisk until combined, 2 minutes. When fully incorporated, pass the coconut cream mixture through a fine mesh strainer set over the bowl with the melted chocolate. Combine with a rubber spatula until thoroughly mixed.

3. In a medium bowl, or in the bowl of a stand mixer fitted with the whisk attachment, whisk the egg white to stiff peaks. Add the honey and whisk again until well combined. Set aside.

4. Fold the egg white mixture into the chocolate mixture, taking care not to overmix. Divide the mixture evenly among four 6-ounce ramekins and refrigerate for at least 4 hours, or until set.

TIP: The custard will keep in the refrigerator covered with plastic wrap for up to 3 days.

Classic Perfect Churros with Cinnamon Sugar

YIELD: 16 CHURROS

Growing up between New York and California, I always loved the feel of a big city, with buzz and excitement around every corner. All the sounds, the people, and the smells! Well, not *all* the smells . . . but definitely the ones of roasted nuts and churros. I have a vivid memory of attending my first Yankees game with my dad and stopping for a warm, perfectly spiced foot-long churro outside the old stadium. That early food memory has inspired me to re-create that beautiful taste and texture, and I'm happy to say I've officially nailed it with this recipe. Don't be intimidated by the choux pastry dough; it is much easier than you think, and so worth the end result. Don't forget, masa harina is corn *flour*. It is not the same as corn meal; don't mix them up!

1 cup water

4 tablespoons unsalted butter (56 grams)

2 packed tablespoons dark brown sugar (27 grams)

½ tablespoon pure vanilla extract (2 grams)

½ teaspoon kosher salt (3 grams)

1 cup all-purpose flour (145 grams)

2 heaping tablespoons masa harina (corn flour) (25 grams)

3 large eggs, at room temperature (150 grams)

Avocado oil, as needed for frying (about 24 fluid ounces)

2 cups granulated sugar (400g)

½ cup ground cinnamon (100g)

1. In a medium saucepan, heat the water, butter, brown sugar, vanilla, and salt over medium-high heat. Cook until butter is completely melted. Add the flour and masa harina and cook, stirring constantly, for 3 minutes, or until the mixture starts to come together into a dough and a film of flour develops on the bottom and sides of the saucepan. Remove from heat.

2. In the bowl of a stand mixer fitted with the paddle attachment, add the dough and let it cool for 3 minutes. With the mixer on medium speed, add the eggs one at a time, waiting for the dough to come back together before adding the next egg. Once all 3 eggs have been added, mix for 1 minute, or until the batter is smooth and shiny.

3. Fit a large pastry bag with a large star tip and transfer the dough to the pastry bag.

4. Add about 2 to 3 inches of oil to a medium, heavy-bottomed saucepan or Dutch oven and attach a candy thermometer securely to the side of the pot. Heat the oil to 375°F.

5. While the oil heats, make the cinnamon sugar by combining the sugar and cinnamon in a medium bowl. Set aside.

6. When the oil reaches 375°F, pipe the churros directly into the hot oil. You want each churro to be 4 to 5 inches long. Use scissors to cut the dough in between piping each churro if needed. Fry the churros in batches of 3 to 4.

7. For soft-chewy churros, cook for 3 to 4 minutes; for soft-firm churros cook for 6 to 7 minutes; and for crispy churros, cook for 8 to 10 minutes. Make sure to flip them halfway through the fry time so they cook evenly.

8. When the churros reach your desired level of doneness, carefully remove them from oil with a spider strainer or heatproof tongs and drop them into the cinnamon-sugar mixture, tossing to coat. Repeat process with the remaining batter and serve immediately.

TIP: These are delicious served with chocolate sauce or dulce de leche! You can also use Strawberry Glaze, Chocolate Glaze, or Maple Glaze (p. 120).

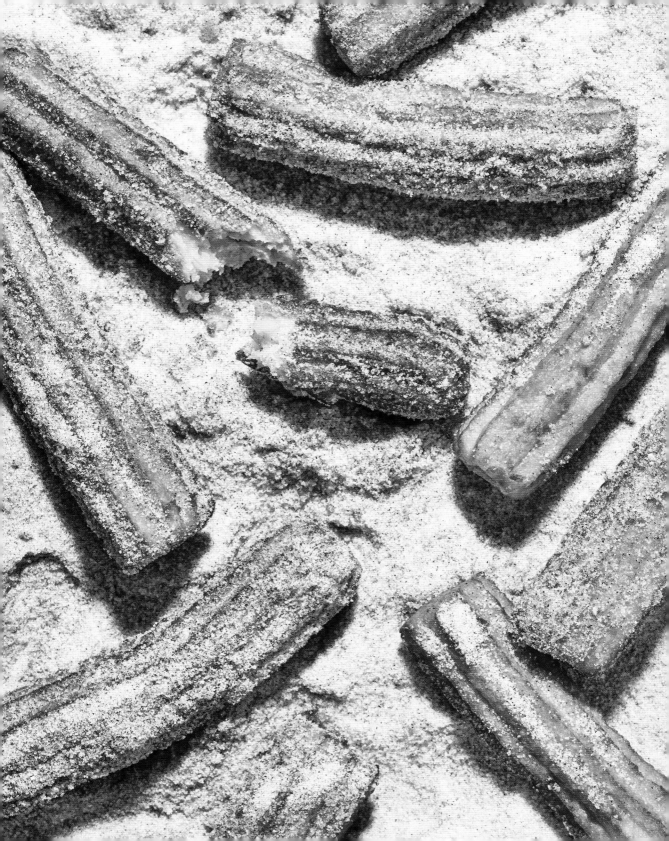

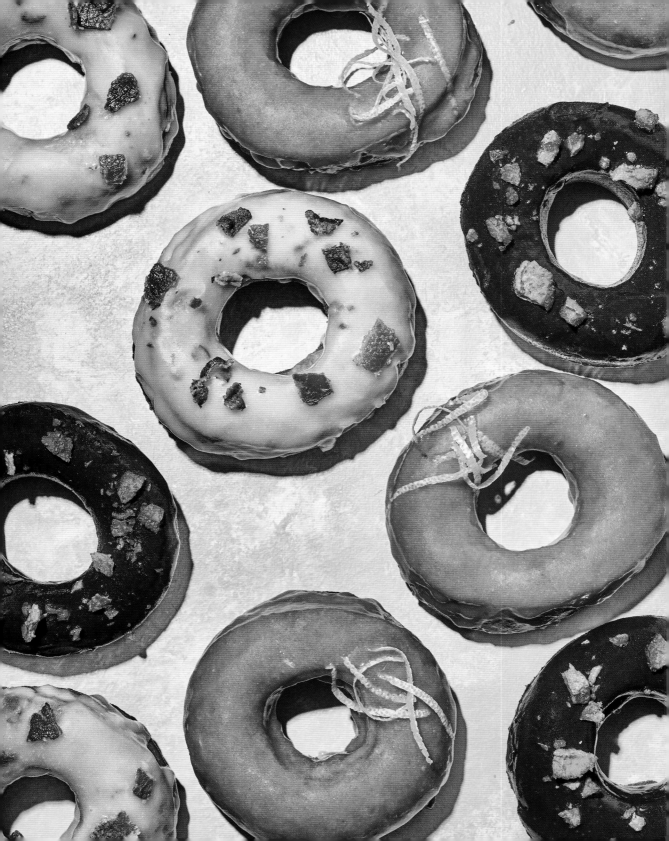

Doughnuts

YIELD: 8 DOUGHNUTS

I love doughnuts with all my heart. When I was a kid, my dad and I would go to Dunkin' to get him coffee, but we'd end up buying a ton of doughnuts . . . such is life. For this recipe, I wanted to offer a few glaze options because I will use any excuse to eat as many doughnuts as possible. Gotta try 'em all, right? Don't be afraid to get creative with your toppings, too. I sprinkle freeze-dried strawberries on the chocolate glaze and shower lemon zest on the strawberry glaze.

¾ cup whole milk (190 grams)

½ cup granulated sugar, divided (100 grams)

1 (¼-ounce) packet active dry yeast (7 grams)

1 large egg (50 grams)

1 large egg yolk (18 grams)

¼ cup (4 tablespoons) unsalted butter, melted (56 grams) plus more for the bowl

½ teaspoon kosher salt (3 grams)

3½ cups bread flour, plus more for dusting (460 grams)

Avocado oil, as needed for frying (about 24 fluid ounces)

Strawberry glaze, chocolate glaze, or maple glaze, for serving (recipes follow)

1. **Make the dough:** In a medium saucepan over medium heat, gently warm the milk to 110°F (it should be warm to the touch, but not hot). Remove from heat, then add ¼ cup of the sugar and all of the yeast to the warm milk and whisk until they dissolve. Allow the mixture to sit until it becomes frothy and the yeast is fully bloomed, 5 minutes.

2. In a large bowl, whisk the egg, egg yolk, and the remaining ¼ cup sugar until light and fluffy.

3. Add the butter and salt to the milk mixture and mix to combine. Then, add the milk mixture to the egg mixture and whisk until fully incorporated.

4. In the bowl of a stand mixer fitted with the dough hook attachment, add the bread flour and milk-egg mixture and knead until the dough comes together. Transfer the dough to a lightly floured surface. Knead by hand for a few minutes until it becomes smooth. Place in a clean, large, greased bowl and cover with plastic wrap. Let the dough rise in a warm place until doubled in size, about 2 hours.

5. After the dough has risen, remove the plastic wrap and gently punch the dough down before kneading it for about 1 to 2 minutes. Return the dough to the bowl, cover it again, and leave it in a warm place for another 45 minutes.

6. Line a baking sheet with paper towels. In a cast-iron skillet or Dutch oven, heat 2 inches of avocado oil over medium-low heat until the oil reaches 350°F. Flour a clean work surface and roll out the dough to about a half inch in thickness and cut out a 4-inch diameter circle using a circular mold or the mouth of a glass, with a small circle cut out in the middle of it as the doughnut hole. Each doughnut should weigh 10 grams. Gently place the doughnut into the hot oil, working in batches to avoid overcrowding the pan. Cook until the doughnuts are golden brown, about 2 to 3 minutes per side. (You can use chopsticks or silicone tongs for turning the doughnuts and taking them out.) Transfer the doughnuts to the lined baking sheet and let cool for a moment before dipping into preferred glaze.

Strawberry Glaze

2 cups hulled strawberries, (140 grams)

5 tablespoons unsalted butter (70 grams)

1 tablespoon heavy cream (10 grams)

¼ teaspoon kosher salt (2 grams)

2 tablespoons fresh lemon juice (20 grams), from 1 small lemon

1 cup confectioners' sugar (130 grams)

1. In the bowl of a food processor or in a high-speed blender, add the strawberries and puree. Strain the pureed strawberries through a fine mesh strainer into a small bowl and set aside.

2. In a medium saucepan, melt the butter over medium heat. Add the pureed strawberries and whisk to combine.

3. Add the heavy cream and salt to the strawberry mixture and stir constantly for about 5 minutes. Remove from the heat and transfer to a heatproof bowl. Whisk in the lemon juice and confectioners' sugar. Cover the glaze with plastic wrap, pressing the plastic to the top of the glaze so a crust doesn't form. Allow the glaze to cool to room temperature before using.

Chocolate Glaze

¼ cup heavy cream (60 grams)

3 tablespoons granulated sugar (37 grams)

¾ cup dark chocolate chips (140 grams)

7 tablespoons unsalted butter (100 grams)

½ teaspoon kosher salt (3 grams)

1. In a small saucepan over medium-low heat, gently warm the heavy cream and sugar.

2. In a double boiler, or in a medium heatproof bowl set over a small saucepan of simmering water (taking care not to let the bowl touch the water), melt the chocolate chips, stirring gently until smooth.

3. Pour the warm cream mixture into the melted chocolate and stir until smooth. Add the butter and continue to stir until completely melted. Add the salt, stir, and remove from the heat. Cover the glaze with plastic wrap, pressing the plastic to the top of the glaze so a skin doesn't form. Allow the glaze to cool to room temperature before using.

Maple Glaze

⅓ cup maple syrup (140 grams)

7 tablespoons unsalted butter (98 grams)

½ teaspoon kosher salt (3 grams)

¾ cup confectioners' sugar (98 grams)

1. In a small saucepan, heat the maple syrup over medium heat.

2. Add the butter and whisk until the butter has melted. Remove from the heat and transfer to a heatproof bowl. Whisking constantly, add the salt and sift the confectioners' sugar. Whisk until fully incorporated. Cover the glaze with plastic wrap, pressing the plastic to the top of the glaze so a skin doesn't form. Allow the glaze to cool to room temperature before using.

NOTE: These glazes can be used not only for the doughnuts, but also with churros (p. 115), funnel cake (p. 99), and beignets (p. 125).

Chocolate Gelato

SERVES: ABOUT 10

Buckle up, because you are in luck with this recipe. The uber-talented Chef Jesse Ventura (my dear friend and the corporate chef of The Herbal Chef) was kind enough to share this recipe that will be the best chocolate gelato you've ever had, guaranteed! The proportions of cream, milk, and chocolate are spot-on, making this absolutely sensational. I highly recommend using the very best milk and cream you can find. Raw milk would be ideal. It makes a huge difference!

8 large egg yolks (125 grams)

½ cup granulated sugar (100 grams)

¾ cup heavy cream (200 grams)

1 cup whole milk (240 grams)

½ teaspoon kosher salt (3 grams)

3½ ounces dark chocolate, chopped (100 grams)

1. In a heatproof medium bowl, add the egg yolks and sugar and whisk until light and fluffy, 3 minutes. Set aside.

2. In a medium saucepan over medium heat, combine the heavy cream, milk, and salt and bring to a simmer. Add the chocolate and stir continuously until it is melted. Add half of the warm cream mixture to the bowl of egg yolks and whisk until combined. Add the egg yolks back to the saucepan with the remaining cream mixture, reduce the heat to medium-low, and cook, stirring constantly with a rubber spatula, until the mixture begins to thicken and can easily coat the back of a spoon, 2 to 3 minutes. Remove from the heat and strain through a fine mesh strainer, then place in an airtight container. Let cool to room temperature, then chill overnight in the refrigerator.

3. Churn the mixture in an ice cream maker according to the manufacturer's instructions. The gelato may be soft after it is first churned, so if you prefer you can let it set up in the freezer for a few hours before serving.

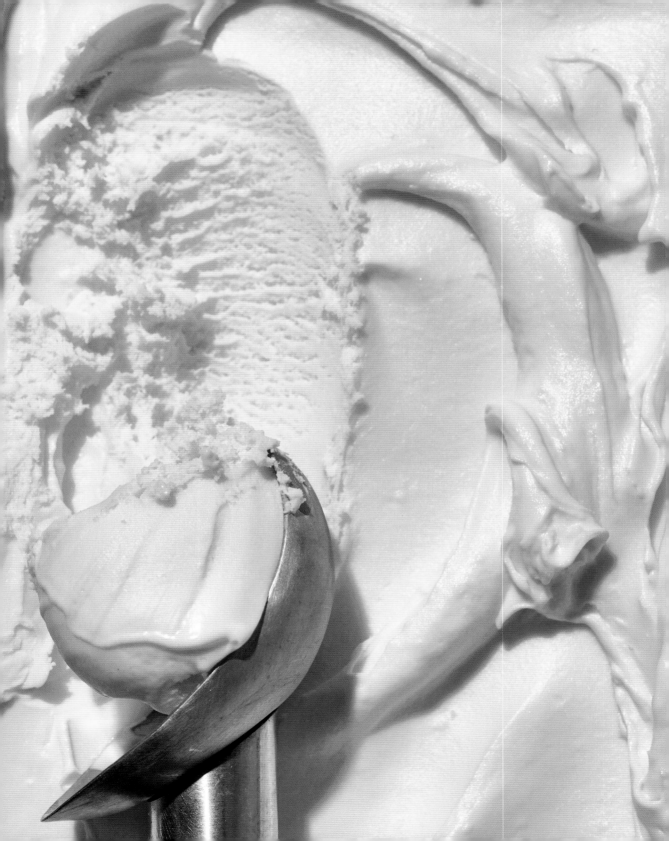

Coconut Gelato

SERVES: 9

This recipe was also created by Chef Jared Ventura. Coconut is my go-to order at gelato shops. The flavor of the coconut drives me . . . well, you get it. This recipe is not one to snooze on, but with a little work up front you can stock your freezer with a batch to last you for weeks! Perfect for a nightcap whenever you want a medicated treat.

8 large egg yolks (144 grams)

½ cup granulated sugar (100 grams)

¾ cup heavy cream (200 grams)

1 cup unsweetened canned coconut milk (237 grams)

½ teaspoon kosher salt (3 grams)

1. In a heatproof bowl, add the egg yolks and sugar and whisk until light and fluffy, 3 minutes.

2. In a medium saucepan over medium heat, combine the heavy cream, coconut milk, and salt. Bring just to a simmer. Add half of the warm cream mixture to the egg yolks and whisk until combined. Add the egg yolks back to the saucepan with the remaining cream mixture, reduce the heat to medium-low, and cook, stirring constantly with a rubber spatula, until the mixture begins to thicken and can easily coat the back of a spoon, 2 to 3 minutes. Remove from the heat and strain through a fine mesh strainer, then place in an airtight container. Let cool to room temperature, then chill overnight in the refrigerator.

3. Churn the coconut mixture in an ice cream maker according to the manufacturer's instructions. The gelato may be soft after it is first churned, so if you prefer you can let it set up in the freezer for a few hours before serving.

Bread Pudding

YIELD: 15 SQUARES

My nonna used to make the most insanely delicious bread puddings for our family when I was a kid. I really wanted to make her proud with this recipe, so I went big on the flavor. The longer this sits in the refrigerator, the better. I call for golden berries here, but if you can't find them, just use some golden raisins or your favorite dried fruit. You can really take creative control with this one!

1 (18-ounce) loaf brioche (460 grams)

6 large eggs (300 grams)

1 cup granulated sugar (200 grams)

½ teaspoon kosher salt (2 grams)

3 cups hemp milk, or any non-dairy milk (720 grams)

1 cup plain whole-milk yogurt (200 grams)

1 teaspoon pure vanilla extract (4 grams)

6 tablespoons unsalted butter, melted, plus more for the pan (84 grams)

1½ tablespoons dark rum (20 grams)

½ teaspoon ground allspice (2 grams)

½ cup dried golden berries (100 grams)

½ cup whole-milk ricotta (110 grams)

1. Preheat oven to 350°F and line two rimmed baking sheets with parchment paper.

2. Cut the bread into 1-inch cubes. Place the bread cubes on the prepared baking sheets and bake until lightly toasted, 10 to 15 minutes.

3. In a large bowl, vigorously whisk the eggs, sugar, and salt together until light and fluffy. Add the hemp milk, yogurt, vanilla, butter, rum, and allspice and whisk until incorporated. Add the toasted brioche to the egg mixture and mix until the bread has absorbed the liquid. Add the dried golden berries and mix to evenly distribute.

4. Grease a 13 × 9-inch baking dish with butter. Spread the mixture into the prepared baking dish and refrigerate for at least 12 hours or up to 24 hours.

5. When ready to bake, preheat the oven to 350°F. Place one rack in the middle of the oven, and place another rack in the upper third of the oven. Make 5 to 10 little pockets with a spoon in the bread pudding and fill them with ricotta. Cover the pan with foil and bake on the middle rack for 35 to 40 minutes, until the bread custard is set.

6. Heat the broiler to high, uncover the custard, and transfer it to the upper rack. Broil until the edges turn golden brown and crispy, 5 to 7 minutes, rotating halfway through. Be sure to keep a close eye on the pudding while it is under the broiler; all ovens vary, so you may only need a minute or two depending on how hot your broiler gets.

Beignets

YIELD: 48 BEIGNETS

When I first arrived in New Orleans, I went straight to Café du Monde and waited forty-five minutes for warm beignets covered in confectioners' sugar. Back at home on the West Coast, I wanted to make something that we could be proud of while still having that nostalgic flavor from the Deep South. These beignets hit the spot. Top them with confectioners' sugar, or you can dip them in dulce de leche or strawberry, chocolate, or maple glazes (page 120) if you're feeling saucy.

¾ cup warm water (110°F) (170 grams)

1 (¼-ounce packet) active dry yeast (7 grams)

2 large eggs (100 grams)

½ cup milk (123 grams)

3 tablespoons unsalted butter, melted (42 grams)

¼ cup plus 2 tablespoons granulated sugar (70 grams)

4 cups bread flour (580 grams), plus more for dusting

½ teaspoon kosher salt (3 grams)

Avocado oil, as needed, for frying (about 24 fluid ounces), plus more for the bowl

Confectioners' sugar, for dusting

1. In a medium bowl, combine the water and yeast. Let stand until foamy, 5 minutes.

2. Add the eggs, milk, butter, and sugar to the yeast mixture and whisk to combine. Set aside.

3. In a large bowl, mix the bread flour and salt. Pour the yeast mixture into the flour mixture, stirring with a spatula to form a loose dough. Turn the dough out onto a clean, lightly floured work surface and knead it with your hands until the dough comes together in a smooth ball.

4. Lightly grease a large bowl with avocado oil. Transfer the dough to the greased bowl and cover tightly with plastic wrap, ensuring the plastic is not touching the dough. Allow the dough to rise in a warm place until doubled in size, 2 hours.

5. After the dough has risen, punch it down, then cover it again and allow to rise for 1 hour more. After the second rise, turn the dough out onto a lightly floured surface.

6. Line a baking sheet with parchment paper. Roll the dough into a large rectangle, about 12 × 16 inches and ½-inch thick. With a sharp knife, cut the dough into 2-inch squares, then transfer the squares to the prepared baking sheet. Set up a wire rack over some paper towels, for draining cooked beignets.

7. In a large pot over medium-high heat, add 2 inches of avocado oil and heat until it reaches 350°F. Working in batches so as not to crowd the pan, carefully lower the dough squares into the hot oil. Fry until golden brown on both sides, 2 to 3 minutes per side. As soon as the beignets puff up, use heatproof tongs to gently flip them over. Transfer the beignets to the wire rack to drain. Dust them with confectioners' sugar and serve warm.

Ice Cream Sandwiches

YIELD: 10 SANDWICHES

I cannot think of a more nostalgic dessert than a classic ice cream sandwich. You know, the ones where the sandwich crumbs stick to your fingers and you have to work a bit to lick off the chocolate? Man, that's the stuff. The ice cream in this recipe can be portioned out with a 2-ounce ice cream scoop or simply put into a circular mold of the same size. I love to make a bunch of these and then store them in the freezer for when my sweet tooth kicks in.

FOR THE COOKIES

4½ cups all-purpose flour (450 grams)

1¾ cups granulated sugar (340 grams)

⅔ cup cocoa powder (70 grams)

1 tablespoon baking powder (12 grams)

½ teaspoon kosher salt (3 grams)

1¼ cups whole milk (308 grams)

½ cup vegetable shortening, melted (140 grams)

2 large eggs (100 grams)

1 teaspoon pure vanilla extract (4 grams)

FOR THE COOKIES & CREAM ICE CREAM

1 large egg yolk (18 grams)

1 cup granulated sugar (200 grams)

3 cups heavy cream (695 grams)

1 cup whole milk (246 grams)

1 teaspoon pure vanilla extract (4 grams)

20 chocolate cookies, crushed into small chunks (150 grams)

1. **Make the cookies:** Preheat the oven to 350°F and line a rimmed sheet pan with parchment paper or a nonstick Silpat.

2. Into a large bowl, sift together the flour, sugar, cocoa powder, baking powder, and salt and whisk to mix. In a separate large bowl, whisk together the milk, shortening, eggs, and vanilla. Add the dry ingredients into the wet ingredients little by little and whisk until combined. Pour the batter in a thin layer on the prepared sheet pan. Bake until slightly risen, 6 to 8 minutes. Set aside to cool.

3. **Make the ice cream:** In the bowl of a stand mixer fitted with the whisk attachment, beat the egg yolk and sugar until light and aerated.

4. In a medium saucepan over medium-low heat, warm the heavy cream, milk, and vanilla to a simmer. Once simmering, add a quarter of the cream mixture to the egg mixture. Whisk until fully incorporated, then add the entire tempered egg mixture back into the saucepan. Cook, stirring continuously, on medium-low heat until the mixture thickens enough to coat the back of a spoon. Cool the mixture on ice, or cool to room temperature before refrigerating overnight, then transfer to an ice cream machine and churn according to the manufacturer's instructions. Fold in the cookie crumbles and pack the mixture into 3-inch circular molds, if using, before putting it in the freezer.

5. **Assemble the sandwiches:** With a cookie cutter, cut circles from the cooled rectangular cookie just slightly larger (about 3.5 inches) than the ice cream molds so you can make a sandwich out of them. Scoop the ice cream on to half of the cookies, then top with the remaining cookies. Wrap each sandwich individually in plastic wrap and freeze. They will keep for about a month.

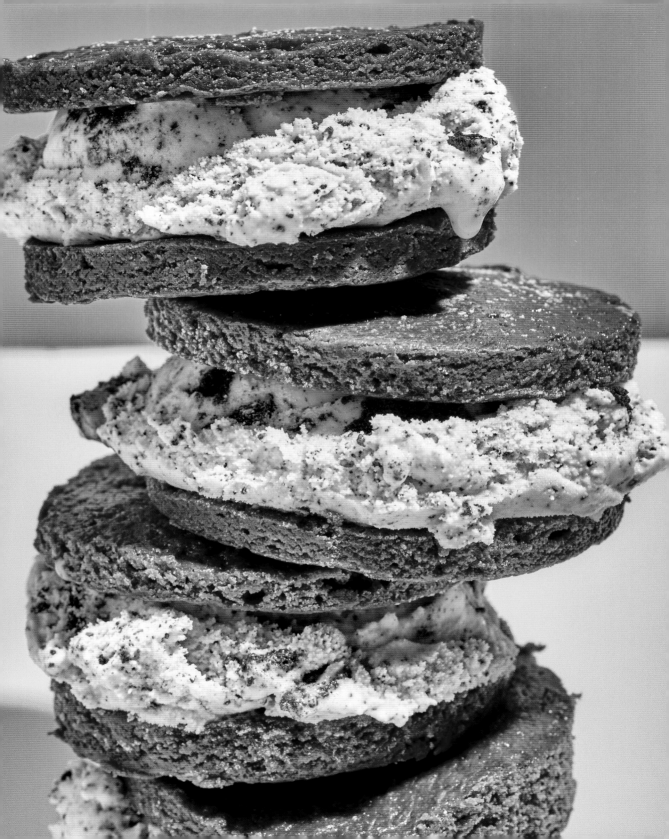

Caramel-Apple Sundaes

YIELD:: 12 SUNDAES

Traditional sundaes are cool and all, but this one is very special: fall flavors in the spiced gelato accompanied by a tart apple caramel and a crunchy nut crumble invented by my friend and colleague Chef Jared Ventura.

FOR THE SPICED GELATO

2¼ cups half-and-half (515 grams)

2 cups granulated sugar (400 grams)

1 tablespoon vanilla bean paste (15 grams)

½ teaspoon kosher salt (3 grams)

¼ teaspoon ground nutmeg

¼ teaspoon ground cinnamon

6 large egg yolks (108 grams)

4 ounces white chocolate, chopped (113 grams)

FOR THE NUT CRUMBLE

¾ cup shelled pecans (100 grams)

⅔ cup whole almonds (100 grams)

¾ cup pepitas (100 grams)

FOR THE APPLE CARAMEL

1 cup granulated sugar (200 grams)

½ cup peeled and diced Granny Smith apple (80 grams)

2 teaspoons vanilla bean paste (10 grams)

2 teaspoons kosher salt (12 grams)

4 tablespoons unsalted butter (56 grams)

½ cup crème fraîche (100 grams)

1. **Make the gelato:** In a medium saucepan over medium heat, add the half-and-half, 1 cup of the sugar, the vanilla bean paste, salt, nutmeg, and cinnamon. Bring to a simmer.

2. In a separate heatproof bowl, whisk the egg yolks and remaining 1 cup of sugar. Add half of the simmering half-and-half mixture to the egg yolks and stir until well combined. Pour the tempered egg yolks back into the saucepan and cook, stirring constantly, until the mixture coats the back of a spoon and reaches 180°F.

3. Prepare a large bowl with ice water and set aside. Add the white chocolate to another clean large bowl. Pour the warm half-and-half mixture over the chocolate, whisking until the chocolate is completely melted. Set the bowl of chocolate inside the bowl with ice water and stir until the contents have cooled to room temperature. Alternately, you can refrigerate the chocolate for at least 2 hours before churning in an ice cream maker per the manufacturer's instructions. Once churned, you may want to chill in the freezer for 3 to 4 hours, or until solid and scoopable.

4. **Make the nut crumble:** Preheat the oven to 350°F. On a large rimmed baking sheet, scatter the pecans, almonds, and pepitas. Toast for 8 to 10 minutes or until very fragrant. Remove from the oven and let cool slightly, then transfer to the bowl of a food processor and process until the mixture resembles coarse sand. Set aside.

5. **Make the caramel:** In a deep medium saucepan, add the sugar, apples, vanilla bean paste, salt, and butter. Cook over medium heat without stirring until the mixture turns an amber color and reaches 225°F, 5 to 6 minutes. Remove from the heat and whisk in the crème fraîche until fully incorporated. Let cool slightly, then add the mixture to a high-speed blender and blend until smooth, taking care as the mixture will expand during the process.

6. In a glass or parfait dish, add a tablespoon of the nut crumble, then drizzle a spoonful of caramel on top to coat the nuts, and top with a scoop of spiced gelato. Repeat with the remaining ingredients and serve immediately.

TIP: When making the caramel, you can gently turn the pot with a flick of the wrist, but you want to allow the sugar to turn amber without stirring it before blending it.

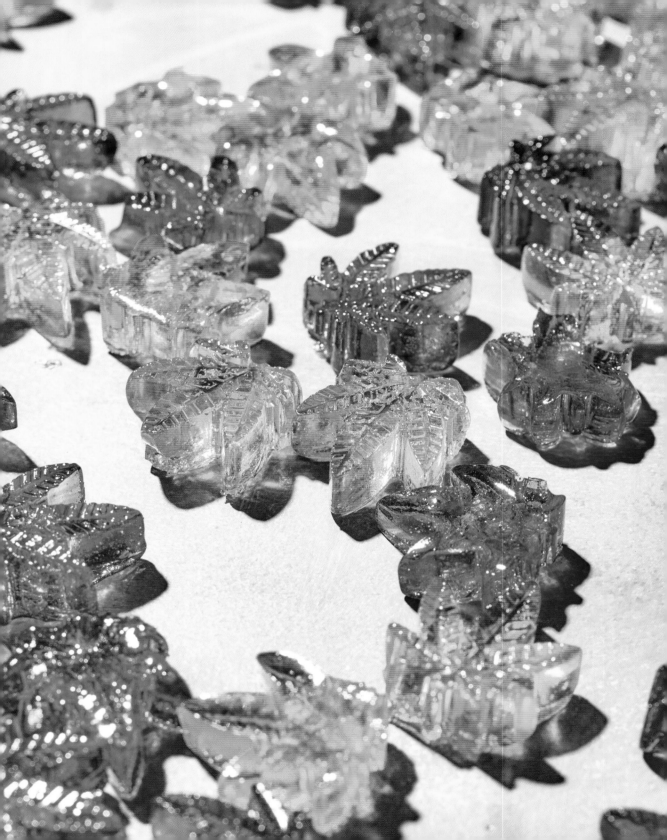

Hard Candies

YIELD: 100 CANDIES
(ABOUT 1G EACH)

In the cannabis industry, hard candies are one of the most sought-after edibles, and for good reason! They are easy to carry around and have a long shelf life. While working with sugar can be a tad intimidating, it's very doable as long as you follow the directions exactly and keep a close eye on both your pot and the candy thermometer. If you do that, these candies will come together easily! Make sure you have all the ingredients and tools you'll need for this at the ready. You don't want to be searching for stuff when you have the sugar boiling away on the stove. LorAnn Oils is my preferred candy flavoring. It is easy to order online.

Nonstick cooking spray, for molds

1½ cups granulated sugar (300 grams)

½ cup inverted sugar or light corn syrup (175 grams)

½ cup water (100 grams)

1 dram LorAnn Oils flavoring of choice

4 to 5 drops LorAnn Oils liquid coloring of choice (optional)

1. Spray candy molds with nonstick cooking spray and set them on a rimmed baking sheet.

2. In a medium saucepan over medium-high heat, combine the sugar, inverted sugar, and water and stir constantly with a heat-safe spatula. Swirl to make sure the liquid heats evenly and doesn't scorch the bottom of the pan. If some sugar crystals stick to the sides of the pan, use a wet pastry brush to scrape the sugar into the pot.

3. Secure a candy thermometer to the side of the pot and cook until the temperature reaches 300°F. Once the sugar mixture reaches temperature, place in a heatproof bowl and add the flavoring, and coloring if using. Mix well with a silicone spatula, then carefully pour into the prepared molds. Use an offset spatula to clean up any spills, working quickly before they set. Let cool completely at room temperature for at least 4 hours, then pop the candies out of molds and store them in an airtight container.

Hand Pies

YIELD: 6 TO 8 HAND PIES

I couldn't make a dessert cookbook that didn't include my all-time favorite childhood snack! Everyone knows these iconic toaster pastries, but this is an easy version that will have you and your friends drooling over the nostalgic treat. I love them served alongside a roaring fire during a movie night with lots of blankets.

FOR THE DOUGH

3¾ cups all-purpose flour, plus more for dusting (468 grams)

1½ cups (3 sticks) unsalted butter, chilled and cut into cubes (336 grams)

4½ tablespoons coconut nectar, also referred to as coconut sap (84 grams)

3 teaspoons kosher salt (18 grams)

3 large eggs (150 grams)

FOR THE MIXED-BERRY FILLING

1 cup mixed berries (blueberries, raspberries, and/or blackberries) (155 grams)

2 tablespoons honey (45 grams)*

2 tablespoons fresh lemon juice, from 1 small lemon (30 grams)

¼ teaspoon kosher salt (2 grams)

1 large egg (50 grams)

1 tablespoon ashwagandha root powder (15 grams), optional inflammatory health benefits

1 teaspoon apple pectin or Further Foods collagen (8 grams) (optional)

FOR THE STRAWBERRY FILLING

1 cup strawberries, hulled and diced (155 grams)

2 tablespoons honey (45 grams)*

2 tablespoons fresh lemon juice, from 1 small lemon (30 grams)

½ teaspoon kosher salt (3 grams)

1 large egg (50 grams)

1 tablespoon ashwagandha root powder (15 grams) (optional)

1 teaspoon apple pectin or Further Foods collagen (8 grams) (optional)

**3 medium Honey Crisp apples,
diced (185 grams)**

3 tablespoons maple syrup
(66 grams)*

**1 tablespoon ground cinnamon
(66 grams)**

**2 tablespoons fresh lemon
juice, from 1 small lemon
(30 grams)**

**¼ teaspoon kosher salt
(2 grams)**

1 large egg (50 grams)

**1 teaspoon apple pectin
or Further Foods collagen
(8 grams) (optional)**

**1 (15-ounce) can coconut
cream**

¼ cup maple syrup (78 grams)

**1 teaspoon vanilla extract
(4 grams)**

**1 tablespoon apple pectin
(15 grams)**

* Add cannabis tincture or
oil and continue with recipe

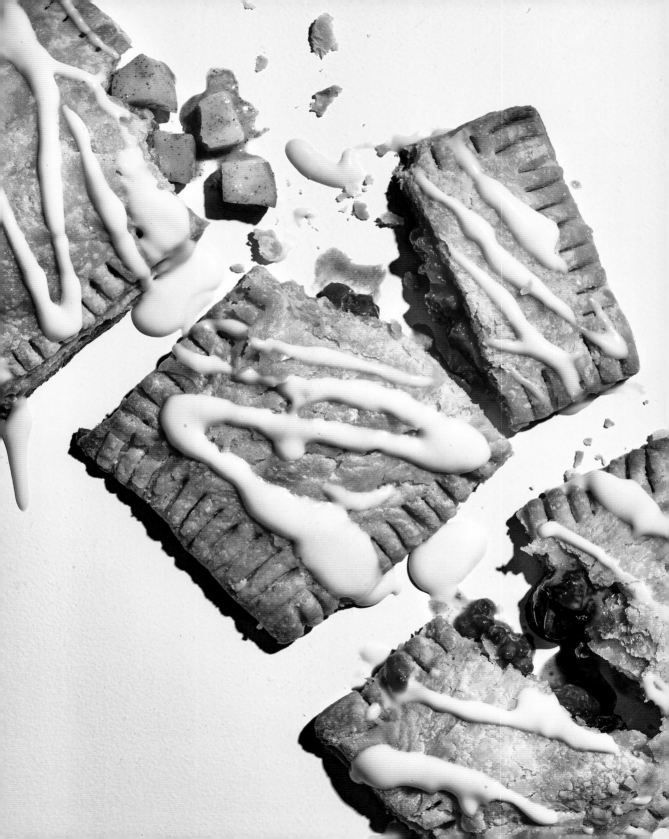

recipe continued

1. **Make the dough:** Into a large bowl, sift the flour and add the butter. Gently work the butter into the flour with a pastry cutter or your hands until it is crumbly.

2. In a small bowl, add the coconut nectar, salt, and eggs and mix well. Add the egg mixture to the flour mixture and knead into a dough. Divide the dough into two large, flat discs and wrap in plastic wrap. Refrigerate the dough for at least 30 minutes, or up to 2 days.

3. Roll the discs between two sheets of lightly floured parchment or wax paper into ¼-inch-thick circles. Cut the dough into uniform rectangles (the size of your hand pies is up to you). Cut "bottoms" and "tops" from the dough, ensuring that the "tops" are slightly larger all the way around to accommodate the filling.

4. **Make the mixed-berry filling:** In a medium saucepan, combine the berries, honey, lemon juice, salt, egg, ashwagandha root power (if using), and apple pectin (if using). Cook over high heat until the filling thickens, 3 to 4 minutes. Remove from the heat and let cool completely before using.

5. **Make the strawberry filling:** In a medium saucepan, combine the strawberries, honey, lemon juice, salt, egg, ashwagandha root powder (if using), and apple pectin (if using). Cook over high heat until the filling thickens, 3 to 4 minutes. Remove from the heat and let cool completely before using.

6. **Make the apple-cinnamon filling:** In a saucepan, combine the apples, maple syrup, cinnamon, lemon juice, salt, egg, and apple pectin (if using). Cook over high heat until the filling thickens, 3 to 4 minutes. Remove from the heat and let cool completely before using.

7. **Assemble the tarts:** Preheat oven to 350°F and line two rimmed baking sheets with parchment paper. Arrange the "bottom" rectangles on the prepared baking sheets. Scoop 1 tablespoon of the desired filling into each "bottom" rectangle. Top each with a "top" rectangle and press the sides together with the tines of a fork. Bake until golden brown, 20 to 25 minutes. Remove and let cool slightly.

8. **Make the icing:** In a medium saucepan over medium heat, combine the coconut cream, maple syrup, and vanilla. Bring to a simmer and add the apple pectin. Transfer the mixture to a high-speed blender (or use an immersion blender) and blend for 1 minute. Return mixture to saucepan and heat over medium heat for 2 minutes more, until the mixture is thick enough to coat the back of a spoon. Allow the icing to cool completely before using. Serve the hand pies immediately after icing.

Pâte de Fruits

YIELD: 64 (1-INCH)
CANDY SQUARES

Gummies are one of the highest-grossing edibles in the entire cannabis market, so I thought I would give you a refined version that has natural ingredients and insanely delicious flavor without the high price tag. I love the passion fruit flavor, but you can use whatever fruit you have. Lastly, the inverted sugar is a specialty item that you can order online, or if you are less particular, you can use corn syrup from the store.

Nonstick cooking spray, as needed

FOR THE PASSION FRUIT PUREE
2½ cups ready-made passion fruit puree (585 grams) (see Tip)

2¾ cups granulated sugar, divided (550 grams)

2 tablespoons apple pectin (30 grams)

2 tablespoons inverted sugar or light corn syrup (40 grams)

⅛ teaspoon cream of tartar

⅛ teaspoon water*

FOR THE COATING
½ cup granulated sugar (100 grams)

1 teaspoon citric acid (10 grams)

* Add cannabis tincture to water and continue with recipe

1. Line an 8 × 8-inch metal pan with plastic wrap, leaving excess on each side so the wrap forms a sort of handle for lifting the gummies out of the pan. Coat the plastic wrap with nonstick cooking spray.

2. In a medium saucepan over medium-high heat, add the passion fruit puree and cook, stirring often with a silicone spatula, until warmed through, about 5 minutes.

3. Meanwhile, in a small bowl, mix ¼ cup of the granulated sugar with the pectin. Add the pectin mixture and inverted sugar to the warm passion fruit puree and whisk until fully incorporated. Add the remaining 2½ cups sugar and whisk to combine.

4. Reduce heat to medium-low. Attach a candy thermometer to the side of the saucepan and cook, stirring often, until the mixture reaches 225°F.

5. While the mixture is coming to temperature, in a small bowl, combine the cream of tartar and water, mixing well so no clumps remain. When the passion fruit mixture reaches 225°F, remove from heat and immediately add the cream of tartar mixture. Whisk to fully incorporate, then pour into the prepared pan.

6. Let it sit at room temperature, covered, for at least 5 hours or overnight.

7. Once set, cut the pâte into 64 equal-size squares, using a scale and a ruler to create even lines and equal portions. In a small bowl, mix the sugar and citric acid together, then coat each square in the mixture, shaking off any excess.

TIP: You can also make the passion fruit puree from fresh passion fruit: Cut 10 to 15 passion fruits in half and scoop out the contents. Strain the flesh through a fine mesh strainer and save the juice and pulp. Blend the juice and pulp with a teaspoon of water until pureed. If you want to use frozen passion fruit, blend passion fruit cubes with 1 tablespoon of water until it's fully smooth.

Chocolate Bonbons

YIELD: 24 SMALL, RICH
BONBONS

I like to serve this CBD-filled treat at the end of a meal, so my guests can enjoy a smooth transition into a euphoric state by combining CBD and THC. I also like to put a nut in the molds, for a little texture. Just make sure to follow the tempering instructions. These truffles also make nice holiday gifts.

FOR THE CHOCOLATE CASING

2½ cups chopped dark chocolate (400 grams), divided

FOR THE GANACHE FILLING

3 cups fresh raspberries (360 grams)

1¾ cups heavy cream (420 grams)

⅓ cup granulated sugar (67 grams)

5 cups chopped dark chocolate (830 grams)

10 tablespoons (1¼ sticks) unsalted butter, at room temperature (140 grams)

1. **Prepare the tempered chocolate casings:** In a double boiler, or in a large heatproof bowl set over a medium saucepan of simmering water (taking care not to let the bowl touch the water), add about 2 cups of the chocolate. Allow it to melt completely and come to 117°F on an instant-read thermometer. Remove from the heat and slowly start incorporating the remaining chocolate (about ½ cup), a few pieces at a time, until the chocolate is fully melted and about 90°F.

2. Pour the tempered chocolate into ¼-ounce chocolate molds, ensuring each mold is fully coated. Invert the mold onto a wire rack set over a sheet pan and let the excess chocolate drip off. Turn upright and use an offset spatula to clean up the edges of the molds, then let set at room temperature for at least 1 hour before filling. Save the excess chocolate in the bowl and keep it at 90°F while stirring occasionally so you can use it to close the shells.

3. **Make the ganache:** In a high-speed blender, add the fresh raspberries and blend until liquid. Strain the raspberries through a fine mesh strainer and discard the seeds. In a medium saucepan, add the raspberry puree, heavy cream, and sugar. Simmer gently over low heat, stirring occasionally, until the sugar is dissolved.

4. Meanwhile, in a double boiler, or in a large heatproof bowl set over a medium saucepan of simmering water (taking care not to let the bowl touch the water), add the dark chocolate. Stir until melted, then remove from the heat and whisk in the raspberry-cream mixture and butter, 1 tablespoon at a time. Transfer to a high-speed blender and blend until smooth. Place the ganache in a piping bag or a sturdy zip-top bag and refrigerate for at least 1 hour, or until firm but pipeable.

5. Once the ganache is somewhat firm, snip the corner of the piping bag. Pipe the ganache into the set chocolate in the prepared molds, leaving some space at the top to add a top layer of tempered chocolate.

6. Top with tempered chocolate and use an offset spatula to clean up the molds. Let sit for at least 1 hour or until the chocolate is completely cooled before unmolding.

TIP: If you are having trouble removing the chocolate from the mold, refrigerate the mold for about 20 minutes and then tap the mold on a firm surface to loosen the truffles.

Cherry-Beet Sherbet

YIELD: 8 SERVINGS

This vibrant sherbet takes me back to days spent at my *jiddeh*'s house in New York when the ice cream truck rolled by. Sometimes I would get the Ninja Turtles or SpongeBob ice pops, but my favorite treat (other than soft serve) was the Flintstones Push Up pop. This recipe is a nod to that childhood favorite but with a bit of a twist from earthy beets and tart-yet-sweet cherries. I highly recommend buying empty push-pop cases to fill with the sherbet. Store the pops in the freezer and pop one out on a hot summer day to feel like a kid again. Alternatively, you can place a 2-ounce scoop of sherbet in separate plastic or glass containers.

1½ cups granulated sugar (300 grams)

⅓ cup plus 2 tablespoons water (100 grams)

2 teaspoons sorbitol (8 grams)

2 cups fresh or frozen pitted cherries (256 grams)

¼ cup diced cooked beets (34 grams)

⅓ cup fresh lime juice (75 grams)

⅓ cup plus 2 tablespoons heavy cream (100 grams)

1. In a small saucepan over medium heat, add the sugar and water and bring to a simmer. Once simmering, remove the saucepan from the heat and measure out 1 cup (200 grams) of the sugar water. Reserve any excess as a sweetener for your favorite beverage. Stir the sorbitol into the syrup to dissolve.

2. In a high-speed blender, add the cherries, beets, lime juice, and sorbet syrup. Blend until smooth. Add the heavy cream and blend until combined. Refrigerate for 1 hour.

3. Once the sherbet has chilled, churn in an ice cream maker according to the manufacturer's instructions. The sherbet may be soft after it is first churned, so if you prefer you can let it set up in the freezer for a few hours before serving. If you are using push-up pop cases, transfer the sherbet to a large piping bag and fill each one. Store in the freezer until ready to serve.

Cucumber Collins (Nonalcoholic)

YIELD: APPROXIMATELY
1 CARBONATED BOTTLE

Some people enjoy a beverage at the end of the evening, and some people enjoy a smoke. This is for the people who like both. The beverage director of The Herbal Chef, Bradley Fry, who really takes his drinks seriously, developed this one, and we wanted to share it with you. A tincture works well in this beverage, which is so delicious and refreshing you might want to double the recipe and make it in batches.

1 ounce apple juice (30 grams)

2 ounces pineapple juice (60 grams)

2 ounces cucumber juice (60 grams)

2 ounces agave syrup (86 grams)

½ ounce fresh ginger juice (8 grams) (see Tip on p. 65)

4 drops saline solution (2 grams)*

2 ounces Seedlip Spice 94 non-alcoholic spirit (60 grams)

* Add cannabis tincture to saline solution and continue with recipe

In a 12-ounce carbonating bottle, such as a Soda Stream, combine the apple juice, pineapple juice, cucumber juice, agave syrup, ginger juice, saline solution, and Seedlip spirit. Carbonate to your taste. If you don't have a Soda Stream or other carbonation device, you can use 4 ounces sparkling water. Serve immediately over ice.

Literally the Best
Hot Chocolate

YIELD: 6 CUPS

I made this recipe for a young woman named Kimber who was battling cancer during the holiday season. We bonded over our love of food. At the time, I wanted to make something delicious she would enjoy, while also supporting her health. This collagen-packed hot cocoa is free of added sugar and dairy (although there is a little bit in the dark chocolate) so it doesn't trigger inflammation. If that is not an issue for you, I would highly suggest making this with raw milk and cream, because the results are outrageous. The frothing is really important in this recipe, too, so don't skip that step!

2 cups almond milk, or plant-based milk of choice (455 grams)

1 teaspoon pure vanilla extract (5 grams)

1 tablespoon chocolate collagen powder (9 grams)

1 (4-ounce) bar 72% dark chocolate, broken into small pieces

½ cup coconut cream (106 grams)

1. In a medium saucepan, combine the almond milk, vanilla, and chocolate collagen powder. Whisk vigorously to incorporate. Place the saucepan over medium-low heat and bring to a simmer.

2. When the milk begins to simmer, add the chocolate pieces one at a time and whisk until the chocolate is fully dissolved.

3. Add the coconut cream to the hot chocolate and whisk again until frothy, velvety, and fully mixed. Divide the hot chocolate among 6 cups and serve warm.

Salted Caramel Chews

YIELD: ABOUT 24 CARAMELS

Chewy caramels have always been one of my favorite sweets. They are the perfect mix of salty, sweet, chewy, and buttery deliciousness. I love to wrap them in cellophane or waxed paper and give them as gifts during the holidays. They will be a big hit with the sweet lovers in your life.

½ cup (1 stick) salted butter (112 grams), softened, plus 2 tablespoons, melted, for the pans

1 cup heavy cream (248 grams)

⅛ teaspoon baking soda

⅛ teaspoon vanilla bean paste, ½ teaspoon pure vanilla extract, or the seeds of ½ dried vanilla bean

¼ teaspoon sea salt

1 cup plus 1 tablespoon granulated sugar (212 grams)

2 tablespoons honey (50 grams)

1. Line a 9 × 13-inch rimmed sheet pan with parchment paper, then brush the entire surface with 2 tablespoons of the butter.

2. In a small saucepan over low heat, combine the heavy cream, baking soda, vanilla, and salt and bring to 122°F to 140°F.

3. In a separate deep, heavy-bottomed stainless steel or copper pot over medium heat, add the sugar and honey and cook without stirring for 9 minutes, or until it turns a deep golden brown, brushing the sides of the pan with a wet pastry brush to prevent crystallization as needed.

4. Stop the cooking of the caramel by adding the butter to the caramelized honey and sugar mixture. It will be slightly bubbling, so be sure to take care when adding the butter.

5. Add the cream mixture to the caramel mixture and place it back over medium heat. Fix a candy thermometer onto the side of your saucepan and cook, stirring continuously, until the mixture reaches 248°F.

6. Remove from the heat and let cool for 30 seconds, then pour onto the prepared sheet pan. Refrigerate for at least 2 hours. Cut into 24 (1 × 2-inch) squares with a sharp knife. Wrap each caramel in cellophane or wax paper.

TIP: To add some texture, you can add toasted crushed nuts after you bring your caramel to 248°F.

Resources

Looking for more information?

Here are some resources that I rely on for information regarding cannabis and its components.

To learn more about the current developments around cannabis, visit the National Library of Medicine for the following study on cannabinoids and health: https://www.ncbi.nlm.nih.gov/pmc /articles/PMC5741114/.

To understand the health effects of cannabis, visit the National Library of Medicine for the following study: https://www.ncbi.nlm.nih.gov/books/NBK425762/.

For information on the current medical knowledge about medical cannabis, please see the following study published by the Mayo Foundation for Medical Education and Research: https://pubmed .ncbi.nlm.nih.gov/30522595/.

To learn more about terpenes, visit Leafly, where you can also find a glossary to break down the terminology behind all things cannabis: https://www.leafly.com/learn/cannabis-glossary/terpenes.

To understand the role of terpenes in human health care, visit the National Library of Medicine for the following study on terpenoids in modern medicine: https://pubmed.ncbi.nlm.nih.gov/18219762/.

For a deep dive into the history of U.S. marijuana prohibition, visit CNBS: The Definitive Online Cannabis Resource: https://www.cnbs.org/cannabis-101/cannabis-prohibition/.

For a guide to consuming cannabis properly, see my in-depth Q&A at https://www.theherbalchef .com/how-to-eat-pot-properly/.

BAKEWARE

For a variety of unique custom molds and ready-to-use stencils, visit MoldBrothers at https://moldbrothers.nl/en/.

To order top-of-the-line kitchen equipment and tools, visit JB Prince at https://www.jbprince.com/.

For innovative vacuum packaging systems, visit https://www.invacus.com/vacuum-packaging -systems.

For high-quality and high-performance scales, visit https://www.edlundco.com/product -category/scales/.

For premium, long-lasting cookware and a range of culinary equipment, visit https://www.matferbourgeatusa.com/ or https://www.breville.com/us/en/home/index.html.

To find innovative bartending tools and accessories, visit https://www.flavourblaster.com/.

For cutting-edge culinary technology that ensures unparalleled precision in cooking temperature, visit https://www.polyscienceculinary.com/.

INGREDIENTS

For some of my recommended baking ingredients, visit https://www.kingarthurbaking.com/ or https://www.bobsredmill.com/.

For my all-time favorite chocolate brand, visit https://www.valrhona-chocolate.com/.

To shop fresh spices and seasonings, visit https://www.spiceology.com/.

For pure vanilla bean paste, visit http://www.nielsenmassey.com)

Other essentials of mine include any brand of avocado oil, unsalted grass-fed butter, or organic free-range chicken eggs.

To shop my favorite candy, gummy-making, and infusion equipment, visit https://www.gummymolds.com/ or https://www.lorannoils.com/. For the health-minded infusion enthusiast, visit https://www.levooil.com/.

I purchase my favorite terpenes at https://www.abstraxtech.com/.
Here are five main factors to consider when choosing cannabis:

1. Freshness: Make sure it isn't stale or overly dried.

2. Aroma: It should smell vibrant and aromatic.

3. Density: Make sure the buds feel nice and full.

4. Organic: Make sure the farms are not using pesticides or chemicals to grow (even if it isn't certified organic).

5. COA: Check for the certificate of analysis (COA) so you know what you are getting is verified.
For a guide to choosing the right strain, visit https://www.cannigma.com/treatment/how-to-choose-a-cannabis-strain-and-is-it-even-possible/.

Here are some of my favorite places to purchase cannabis:

For online delivery, visit https://www.eaze.com/.

To purchase from farms/dispensaries, visit https://www.sherbinskis.com/ or https://ember-valley.com/.

For delivery in California, visit https://www.urbananow.com/ or https://www.goe.menu/.

Notes

1   Betsy Pearl, "Ending the War on Drugs: By the Numbers," Center for American Progress, June 27, 2018, https://www.americanprogress.org/article/ending-war-drugs-numbers/.

2   Aidan J. Hampson, Julius Axelrod, and Maurizio Grimaldi. Cannabinoids as antioxidants and neuroprotectants. US Patent 6630507-B1, filed April 21, 1998, and issued October 7, 2003.

3   Ethan B. Russo, "Taming THC: Potential Cannabis Synergy and Phytocannabinoid-Terpenoid Entourage Effects," *British Journal of Pharmacology* 163, no. 7 (August 2011): 1344–64, https://doi.org/10.1111/j.1476-5381.2011.01238.x?.

Metric Charts

The recipes that appear in this cookbook use the standard US method for measuring liquid and dry or solid ingredients (teaspoons, tablespoons, and cups). The information on these pages is provided to help cooks outside the United States successfully use these recipes. All equivalents are approximate.

Metric Equivalents for Different Types of Ingredients

A standard cup measure of a dry or solid ingredient will vary in weight depending on the type of ingredient. A standard cup of liquid is the same volume for any type of liquid. Use the following chart when converting standard cup measures to grams (weight) or milliliters (volume).

STANDARD CUP	FINE POWDER (ex. flour)	GRAIN (ex. rice)	GRANULAR (ex. sugar)	LIQUID SOLIDS (ex. butter)	LIQUID (ex. milk)
1	140 g	150 g	190 g	200 g	240 ml
¾	105 g	113 g	143 g	150 g	180 ml
⅔	93 g	100 g	125 g	133 g	160 ml
½	70 g	75 g	95 g	100 g	120 ml
⅓	47 g	50 g	63 g	67 g	80 ml
¼	35 g	38 g	48 g	50 g	60 ml
⅛	18 g	19 g	24 g	25 g	30 ml

Useful Equivalents for Dry Ingredients by Weight

(To convert ounces to grams, multiply the number of ounces by 30.)

OZ	LB	G
1 oz	1/16 lb	30 g
4 oz	¼ lb	120 g
8 oz	½ lb	240 g
12 oz	¾ lb	360 g
16 oz	1 lb	480 g

Useful Equivalents for Length

(To convert inches to centimeters, multiply the number of inches by 2.5.)

IN	FT	YD	CM	M
1 in			2.5 cm	
6 in	½ ft		15 cm	
12 in	1 ft		30 cm	
36 in	3 ft	1 yd	90 cm	
40 in			100 cm	1 m

Useful Equivalents for Liquid Ingredients by Volume

TSP	TBSP	CUPS	FL OZ	ML	L
¼ tsp				1 ml	
½ tsp				2 ml	
1 tsp				5 ml	
3 tsp	1 Tbsp		½ fl oz	15 ml	
	2 Tbsp	⅛ cup	1 fl oz	30 ml	
	4 Tbsp	¼ cup	2 fl oz	60 ml	
	5⅓ Tbsp	⅓ cup	3 fl oz	80 ml	
	8 Tbsp	½ cup	4 fl oz	120 ml	
	10⅔ Tbsp	⅔ cup	5 fl oz	160 ml	
	12 Tbsp	¾ cup	6 fl oz	180 ml	
	16 Tbsp	1 cup	8 fl oz	240 ml	
	32 Tbsp (1 pt)	2 cups	16 fl oz	480 ml	
	64 Tbsp (1 qt)	4 cups	32 fl oz	960 ml	
			33 fl oz	1000 ml	1 L

Useful Equivalents for Cooking/Oven Temperatures

	FAHRENHEIT	CELSIUS	GAS MARK
FREEZE WATER	32°F	0°C	
ROOM TEMPERATURE	68°F	20°C	
BOIL WATER	212°F	100°C	
	325°F	160°C	3
	350°F	180°C	4
	375°F	190°C	5
	400°F	200°C	6
	425°F	220°C	7
	450°F	230°C	8
BROIL			Grill

Acknowledgments

I sure have a lot of people to thank: my family, my dear friends, and my incredible team at The Herbal Chef, who were kind enough to support me throughout the process of writing this book. I love you all. Your encouragement and guidance throughout the process has been a blessing. I also would like to thank all those who have been cheering The Herbal Chef from the sidelines and sending positive messages. You have no idea how much I appreciate that, and without you this book would not be possible. A big thank you to Jake Zidow, whose framework allowed me to take cannabis cuisine to new heights.

Thank you, Natasha, for believing in me and making this book a reality, in addition to Molly and Sara for all the recipe testing. Lastly, thank you to my awesome editor, Doris.

Index

Ingredients that contain infusions are indicated by italicized page numbers.

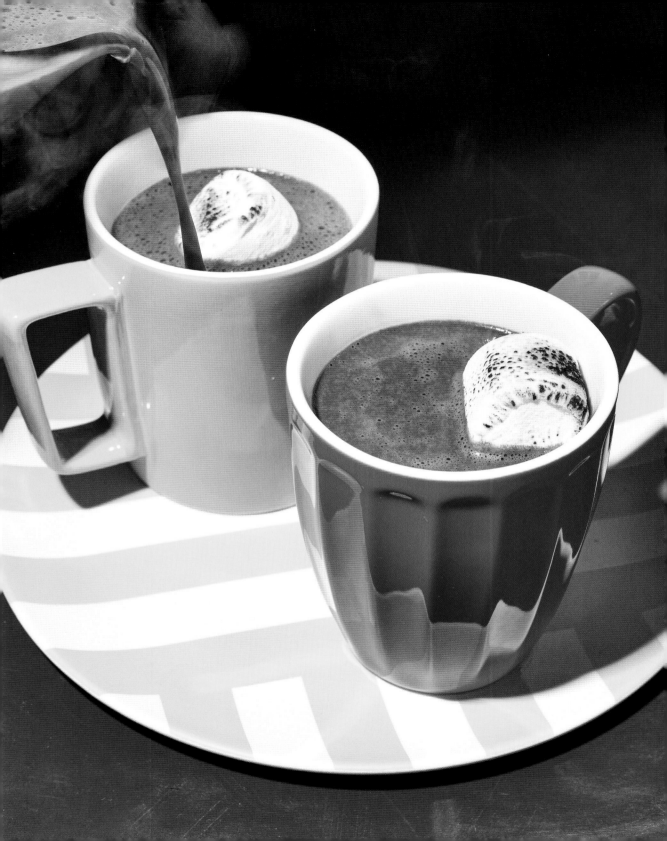

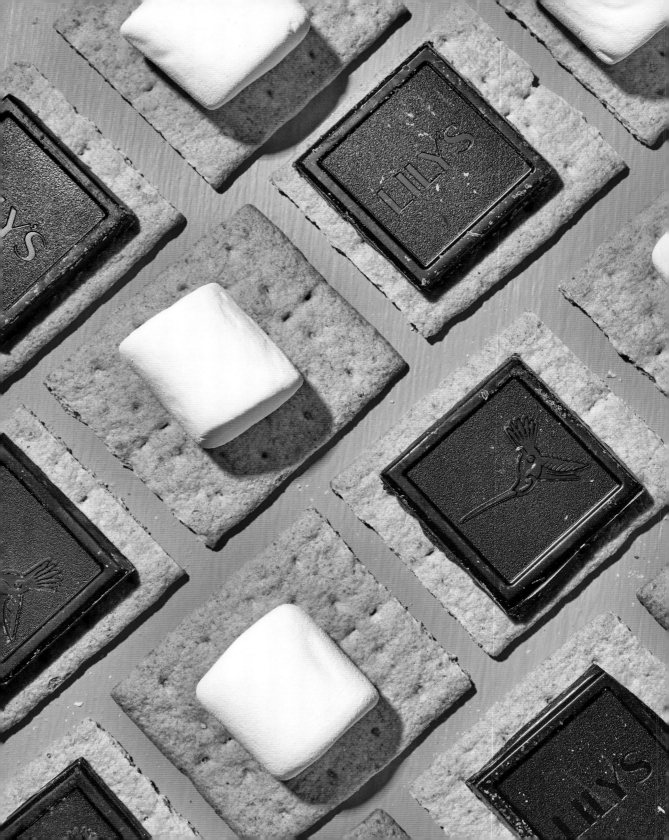

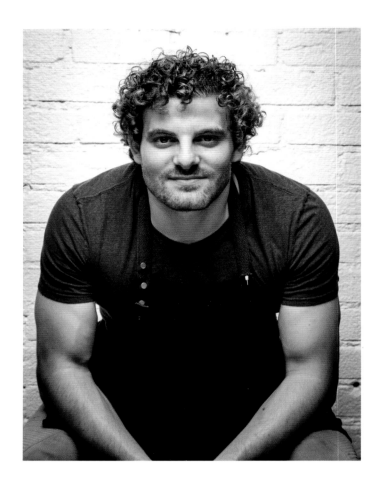

About the Author

Chris Sayegh is the founder and CEO of The Herbal Chef™, a
leading plant medicine hospitality platform with brick-and-mortar stores
in Santa Monica, California. A passionate science and biology student
who turned to the chemistry of food plant medicine, Sayegh was among
the first culinary professionals to enter the cannabis industry and has
pioneered cannabis-infused fine dining in an effort to destigmatize and
elevate the perception of marijuana and other plant medicines. He is
a consultant to the National Restaurant Association, and his work
launching and growing The Herbal Chef has been featured in *GQ*,
Forbes, *Fast Company*, and on CNN, Fox News, and CBS.